Does *IT* wet the bed?

A memoir

Aideen Blackborough

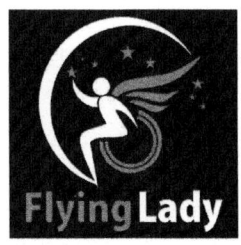

Does *IT* wet the bed?

Copyright © Aideen Blackborough 2015

Photos copyright © Aideen Blackborough

This print edition published 2015 by Flyinglady

First published August 2015 as an eBook by Flyinglady

www.flyinglady-training.com

The moral right of Aideen Blackborough as the author of this work has been asserted in accordance with the Copyright, Designs and Patents Act 1988

Edited by Norman Lindsey

ISBN-13: 978-1515169383

The publisher has no responsibility for the persistence or accuracy of URLs for external or third-party internet websites referred to in this book, and does not guarantee that any content on such websites is, or will remain, accurate or appropriate.

Acknowledgements

Writing the book has been an extremely emotional experience, almost like looking through an old family album. I've laughed and cried as memories have flooded back to me. I've chatted to friends and family about various events that have happened and sometimes been amazed by how their recollections of things have differed from mine. These conversations have led me to do quite a bit of rewriting and I'd like to thank them all for their valuable input into this book.

When I was born, my parents knew very little about cerebral palsy. They just had to take every day as it came and I know the future seemed quite uncertain for them. Without their strength and utter determination to get me into mainstream education, I definitely wouldn't be where I am today. I owe them a lifetime of thanks for everything they have done. I'd also like to thank them for doing their best for 'filling in the gaps' while I've been writing this book. Although my memory is pretty good, many of the recollections of my early childhood have been helped by Mum and Dad. As may be expected, their perceptions of things have occasionally differed and at times, it's been difficult to establish exactly when and why particular things have happened. But I've tried to be as detailed and accurate as I possibly can be.

My family have always offered endless amounts of encouragement and have of course played a central role in my story. I am so lucky to have a family who willingly embraced my disability, as well as all its challenges. Mum, Dad, my dear sisters Collette and Martina and my 'little' brother, James: all the thanks in the world will never seem enough.

I'd particularly like to sincerely thank my best friend, Brian, who has helped me with the initial editing of the book and the cover design. He's always been a brilliant sounding board and never shied away from constructive criticism! Thanks to another critical friend, Graeme Duffy, who was the first to clap eyes on my first draft. He made some sound and valuable suggestions which helped shape the book into what it is today.

Also another dear friend, Mary Mac, has offered endless cups of coffee as I've pondered over the book. Another great sounding board!

My trusted editor, Norman Lindsey, has done a fantastic job of guiding me in the right direction, never *telling* me what to do but steering me towards the right decisions. He's advised on many aspects of the book, not just the text and I have enjoyed working with him so much!

Finally, thanks to my husband Dean. He's kept me motivated whenever I felt like giving up; talked through endless ideas with me and pushed me just to keep writing until I had something worth sharing. I don't think I'd have a book without him! And I mustn't forget our little boy, Jack. You're the absolute sunshine of my life and have afforded the book with a wonderful ending. I love you to the moon and back, Jack.

Contents

Prologue. . .

1. Just lazy
2. Battle lines drawn
3. True Grafters
4. Does *it* wet the bed?
5. If at first you don't succeed. . .
6. A local celebrity
7. Speaking up for myself
8. Head down and mouth shut
9. Summer of '97
10. Another battle
11. Torn
12. Fifteen minutes of fame
13. Flying the nest
14. Burnt pasta bake
15. Two sheets to the wind
16. Suited and Booted
17. Commuting hell
18. Kindness of strangers
19. Sixty-one point three
20. Me, myself and I
21. Free-wheeling
22. All dolled up
23. "Bit wobbly on my feet"
24. Bag of nerves
25. Cloud nine
26. A friendship lost

27. An Irish Tradition
28. Flyinglady
29. The green light
30. Two pink lines
31. One strong, regular heartbeat
32. Morning, noon and night
33. Not quite right
34. Absolutely gorgeous
35. We'll see!

. . . Afterword

Prologue

The day had dawned and it was hard to believe, like waking from an amazing dream, expecting to be catapulted into reality with a bump. But it doesn't happen. Today is *really* happening and it's my dream come true.

I'd always exceeded people's expectations of me, always surprised them with my intelligence and hidden abilities. They took one look at me and expected very little...

I wasn't looked upon as a *normal* child. They said, 'You can't...', but I just shrugged and said, 'Watch me!' I was written off as some kind of invalid, a drain on society just because I have cerebral palsy.

My disability has always been irrelevant to me - it hasn't held me back or stopped me fulfilling all of my dreams. Over the years, people have often asked me if I wished things had been different, or if I would prefer to be able bodied. And the simple answer is no. My life wouldn't be what it is today if I didn't have cerebral palsy. And that's the point – I have cerebral palsy. *It* doesn't have me.

I had already proved that disability didn't equal inability; today I was proving that disability doesn't exclude normality. Today, I was getting married.

Chapter 1
Just lazy

I'm the third of four children and have two older sisters, Collette and Martina, and a 'little' brother, James. I was due to be born at the end of April 1983, but I was late – which is so ironic as I hate being late for anything!

At the time of my birth, my parents were living in County Sligo, Ireland. My Mum went to Sligo General Hospital on 6 May as she was concerned that I hadn't made my appearance yet. The midwives didn't seem overly concerned and she was given drugs to induce labour. Unfortunately, Mum was given an overdose and the staff failed in their duty to monitor Mum or me. They didn't realise that I was in distress and their negligence was to have an impact for the rest of my life.

After a very difficult birth, I was obviously very distressed and upon delivery I wasn't breathing. A doctor as well as an oxygen tank had to be located and it was 25 minutes before I was able to breathe independently. It was during this time that the irreversible damage was done to my brain that caused my cerebral palsy - although of course, nobody realised at the time.

My Dad witnessed all of this and I cannot imagine my parents' relief when I finally began to cry.

Although obviously traumatised by the events of that day, my parents were assured that I was a normal, healthy child and so took me home to 13 Cartion Heights, County Sligo. (Dad is a little superstitious and from that day to this, he won't have anything to do with the number 13 as he's convinced it caused bad luck.) Already having my two sisters, my parents were by now pros – they were familiar with what was normal child development and all the milestones that I should be reaching. But as the months went by, they realised I wasn't doing things as quickly as my sisters had. I was quite 'floppy' and by six months of age, I still couldn't sit up by myself and I didn't start walking until I was gone two. I don't think I was a particularly happy baby either, but that could have just been me being a bit of a madam! Mum tells me that she used to beg Collette and Martina to take me out in my pram just so she could get some jobs done. But her peace was always short-lived as my sisters would quickly return home when I failed to be subdued!

Nonetheless, my parents knew something wasn't right but they just couldn't put their finger on what was wrong. At this stage, the doctors that I had seen had failed to come up with a diagnosis. Despite my parents' concerns that I wasn't reaching the usual childhood milestones, the medical professionals assumed that I was just a lazy child and I would catch up. But this didn't sit right with my parents. I guess what they say is true though – nobody knows your child like you do and my parents knew it was more than just laziness on my part.

It wasn't until my parents decided to emigrate to Australia, that they discovered I might have cerebral palsy (CP). I'm told that we were pretty much set to go, but before we would be allowed into Australia, we all had to undergo a medical examination. Unfortunately, I failed my medical and our application was rejected. The Australian Doctor who had dealt with our application explained to my parents. Dad remembers being totally confused as he had never heard about CP and the doctor failed to elaborate on what it meant. Neither he nor Mum knew anything about the condition or its implications for my future. But it did confirm their fears that my slow development was down to something more serious than *'just laziness'*.

Although naturally disappointed that we had being excluded from emigrating to Australia, I think in a way it was a blessing as this spurred my parents on to get a proper diagnosis. Some time later Mum took me to the hospital for one of many appointments. It was just me and Mum when my own consultant finally felt able to diagnose me. Although Mum had her suspicions and had had them for quite some time, I think it still came as a shock to finally have it confirmed. Mum tells me that the doctor referred to my condition as being spastic – in those days that was the accepted terminology and I think Mum knew what it meant, even if she didn't yet realise the effect it would have on my life.

The term *cerebral* refers to the brain, which is affected by damage caused before or during birth. The word '*palsy*' refers to disorder of movement, or in other words, tremors of any number of body parts including hands, legs, arms or the whole body.

One definition of the condition is, 'a persistent (but not unchanging) disorder of movement and posture, as the result of one or more non-progressive abnormalities in the brain, before its growth and development are complete. Other clinical signs may be present as well.' (www.patient.co.uk)

Cerebral palsy is different for everyone – there are no hard or fast rules but there are three main types of the condition. Some people with CP have one type, while others may have elements of all three. The most common type of CP is ataxia, which basically means 'a lack of muscle coordination when performing voluntary movements.' (National Institute of Health, 2011). The second type is called spasticity, which causes stiff or tight muscles and exaggerated reflexes. Although the definitions refer to the muscles, it is the part of the brain that controls the muscles which causes the difficulties – not the actual muscles themselves. I have a mix of both ataxia and spasticity and know relatively little about the third type which is referred to as dyskinetic CP. According to the Reeve Foundation (www.christopherreeve.org), this type affects 10-20% of people who have CP and it affects the entire body. This type is characterised by fluctuation in muscle tone which is either too tight or too loose.

Cerebral palsy is most often caused by a lack of oxygen to the brain at birth or an accident during early childhood. CP isn't hereditary and it can't just be 'developed' – it occurs after birth and may not be diagnosed for some months or even years later. Its severity is extremely varied and as I said, CP is different for everyone and I don't think I've ever met anyone who experiences it in the exact same way that I do. Some people have very little movement and use a wheelchair full-time, others have very mild symptoms and have never needed a wheelchair. I'm somewhere in between – I use my electric wheelchair outdoors and for long distances but when I'm at home, I am able to and prefer to walk around to try and keep a level of mobility.

But back then, when Mum got that first diagnosis some thirty years ago, it was a condition that was heard of, but oddly not well known. I can only imagine Mum's confusion and upset as we drove home. She finally had confirmation of what she'd suspected all along. I wasn't just a lazy child, I had a long-term disability, which would affect me for the rest of my life. But to this day, I am angry that the doctor broke this news to my Mum when she was alone – he must have realised the enormous effect it would have and Dad wasn't even there.

There was no internet back then and access to information was poor – my parents just had to take every day as it came. But to them, I was just Aideen. Their third daughter who would just need a little extra support. From that day, they were absolutely determined that I wouldn't be treated any differently, either at home or by the world outside. If I was naughty, I still got told off and believe me, I was no angel! My baby album shows me as a mischievous three year old sitting on the stairs, picking off the wallpaper! Mum mustn't have liked that wallpaper too much though, as rather than tell me off, she took the photo!

Now that my parents and the doctors knew that I had cerebral palsy, they were able to start thinking about what lay ahead. I was slow to start walking and so when I was three, my consultant recommended an operation which would help me to stand and walk a little bit straighter. A bone would be removed from my leg and then inserted back into my ankle so that my foot would be better positioned for walking. It was the first of many interventions to try and lessen the impact that CP would have on me and the hospital stay is one of my earliest memories. I can still remember the small single room that I was in, right opposite the nurses' station. I had lots of visitors and I remember two in particular who came from our church. I could hardly see them as they entered the room with a huge cuddly toy for me! I wasn't a bit concerned about being in hospital if I was being so spoilt!

It was still early days following my diagnosis and I think my parents were keen to try anything which had the potential to make life easier for me. They were always determined that I wouldn't end up in a wheelchair full-time and I am incredibly grateful for their resolve. The operation was successful and made me much more mobile. Although I wasn't all that steady, this early intervention ensured that I would have some level of mobility.

I was in a cast up to my knee for about a month, but that didn't seem to bother me. Shortly after my operation, we went to visit my aunt and uncle who were based in Germany with the Army. Even in my cast, I had great fun flying down the toboggan run with my cousins, always begging for another go when we reached the bottom! I was born a dare devil!

By this time, we had moved from Sligo and had settled in Great Barr, Birmingham. When my parents made the decision to move back to the UK (where they had lived for a time previously), they were unaware of my condition and so the decision wasn't based on my needs. Nonetheless, I think it proved wise in the long run. As much as Ireland will always be home to me, I'm not sure the education system in Ireland back then would have given me the good start I had over here.

When I was two, I started at the Toy Library in Dudley, Stourbridge – a nursery school for special needs children. It was started in 1979 and aimed to help children '…in the form of therapeutic, educational and stimulating toys and equipment…' It was a fair trek from our home in Great Barr, but the main reason my parents sent me there was because they provided excellent speech and language therapy which I needed to help my speech before starting school. Obviously, I don't remember much of my time at the Toy Library except that my Uncle Ron, one of my Mum's brothers would regularly collect me and take me to the nearby Zoo! Uncle Ron and I were close as I grew up, always having great fun and if I was very lucky, Uncle Ron would take me to the pub on the way home – yes I know, I started young!

My parents always saw the Toy Library as a

stepping stone to getting me into mainstream education. In their mind, there was never any question about it. As Mum always said, I had as much right to an education as any other child and she was absolutely determined that I'd be given that opportunity.

However, the Local Authority had very different ideas. They felt that I would be a strain on resources, hold the other children back and never achieve anything. So they wanted to send me to a 'special school' for disabled children. Even then, my parents knew I was capable of more and refused point blank to send me to an institute. They knew I'd be put in a wheelchair in front of a TV and never learn anything. They had made up their minds that I was going to the local Roman Catholic (RC) primary school and so their fight to get me a place and then keep me there began: and it didn't end until the day I left.

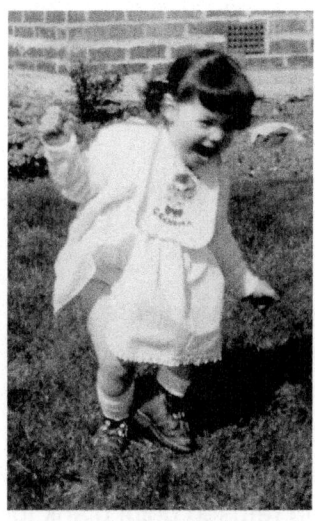

I was almost two when I started walking.

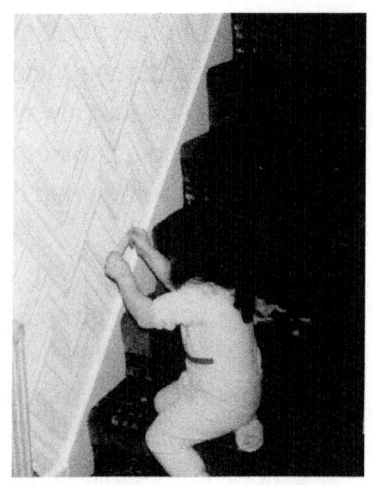

Mum and Dad didn't want me to be treated any differently, although on this occasion, the photo came before the telling off!

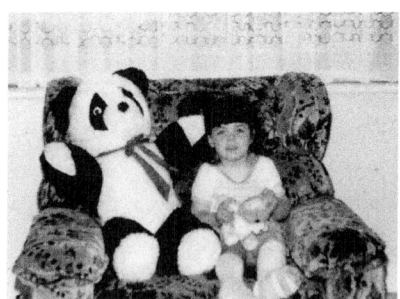

My operation was the first of many interventions to try and ease the impact that CP would have on me.

Chapter 2
Battle lines drawn

The local primary school had an excellent reputation, with some of the best results in the area and this was largely down to the Head Teacher. She was a rather serious lady who ran a very tight ship, commanding much respect from her pupils and parents alike. There was no doubt that her school was the best that I could have gone to, but back then many held the view that segregation worked best, so there was little point in rocking the boat. I have little doubt that the Head had probably never encountered such a situation before and was only thinking of what was best for the school when she resisted my placement.

But my parents were adamant that I should be afforded exactly the same opportunities as any other child. They had been told that the Local Authority were obliged to provide funding to enable me to participate in mainstream education. And so, after several meetings and no doubt some quite heated discussions with the authorities, I was eventually granted a place at the school on the condition that I was supported by a nursery nurse, so that I didn't demand too much of the teacher's time. Little did they know how intelligent I was and that years later, I would graduate with a 2.1 honours degree from Oxford Brookes University. Not that I'm a big head or a told-you-so kind of person, of course!

But my parents didn't care – as long as I was allowed a mainstream education like everyone else, they were happy. However, I remember many frustrating days when my nursery nurse was ill or on training, I wouldn't be allowed to go to school. It was upsetting, as in my mind I was just the same as the other kids and I absolutely loved going to school. But I understand that the Head had to minimise disruption to the other children and perhaps also listen to any concerns raised by the teachers. Although I was aware that my place at the school was always ambivalent, I always felt included by the teachers. Just like at home, I was treated the same as the other kids and I think it soon became apparent that despite my physical limitations, I had no such intellectual barriers. I loved school and thrived from day one.

Nonetheless, I was always aware of my parent's ongoing battle to keep me in the school and I remember one particular evening when the Head and a fellow teacher visited our house to discuss my future with Mum and Dad. At this stage, I must have been in Year One or Two, I had settled in well and I was more than keeping up with my classmates. I don't really know the reasons for that particular meeting, but I can only speculate that the Head was trying to run the school to the highest of standards with limited resources and my presence in the school presented additional challenges. She wanted to appeal to my parents to reconsider my future and give thought to sending me to the local specialist school.

I have a vague memory of being upstairs in my room, I knew the Head was there and as the conversation progressed, it became quite heated. My parents were adamant – I had as much right to a mainstream education as any other child and I was staying in the school. I was doing so well, what reason was there to move me? Especially as I'd be moved to a special school and all the progress I'd made up until now would be ignored and wasted. However, the Head was no doubt facing her own predicaments and was feeling under pressure to provide the best education that she could for the other children. She also felt that my needs would be better met in the specialist school. But this was an argument the Head wasn't going to win. She left our house with the issue unresolved.

This was the constant battle that my parents faced – from one day to the next, they didn't know whether my place at the school would remain. I was aware of this ongoing struggle but despite this, I continued to flourish at school. I definitely had the potential to do well and with the support of my nursery nurse, I participated in everything that my classmates did – including the annual sports days. One particular year, I remember being given a head start in one of the races. I was so slow and unsteady, nobody expected it to make much of a difference. But I think by now, you're realising what a determined madam I was, right? Yes, you've guessed correctly – I came first! I had won a race and nobody could believe it! I was so chuffed with myself, I dismissed the tiny detail of the head start.

Looking back on it now, the eighties was the time when disabled people (and their families) started pushing for a change in attitude, when the Social Model of Disability started to stand up to the older Medical Model. But it would take a long time to percolate into mainstream educational thinking. My parents knew me inside out, they knew that my disability would never be a barrier to me fulfilling my potential. Rightly or wrongly, society just accepted that segregation worked – it was only disabled people and their families who knew better.

As I've said before, my parents never looked at me and saw a disabled child who needed to be cured. They just saw me – their third daughter, Aideen, who they believed had the same potential to achieve as any other child and although they didn't realise it at the time, they were becoming advocates for the Social Model of Disability. They were absolutely determined that I wouldn't be hidden away and forgotten about – hence their long battle to keep me in mainstream education.

Despite the ongoing battle to keep me in the school, I generally got on well with all of my classmates. I had two "best" friends - Lynsey and Linzi. The names got quite confusing at times, but the three of us spent all our break times together and were always at each other's houses for tea. Other kids came and went, but the three of us always stuck together and it was great to be part of a group.

And then there was Austin. I'm sure he won't mind me saying that Austin was a bit of a rogue, all be it a loveable one! He became extremely protective of me and although I used to pretend to be disgusted when Austin insisted on kissing me smack on the lips, I always knew he'd do anything for me and one day, he proved that to his detriment.

Austin was in the playground and he must have overheard one of the other kids making fun of me. Austin wasn't about to ignore it – he got into a punch-up with this kid and landed himself an abrupt trip to the Head's office. But Austin was far from remorseful. He was protecting me no matter what and even our scary Head couldn't extract an apology from him! I think he got a good telling off and a detention for what he'd done but it didn't faze him. He always used to tell me he'd do anything for me and from that day, I believed him!

I generally got on well with all of my classmates, with just one exception – Scarlett. She used to hang around with me and my friends, but I always felt, even then, that she was looking down her nose at the rest of us. Being the youngest in her family, Scarlett perhaps usually got what she wanted. I remember one particular spat with her in the playground. She had somehow persuaded me to lend her one of my favourite books and although reluctant, I wasn't a selfish child and thought it only right to share. But when Scarlett returned the book, a page had been torn out of it. It was my favourite book and Scarlett knew that, yet she hadn't bothered to look after it and even denied that she'd done anything wrong. Normally a happy, easy going child, I was furious and it signalled the start of a feud between us which bubbled away until we left Holy Name. Funny how you remember these silly little things over twenty years later, but some people just rub you up the wrong way I suppose!

Although in many ways, I was just the same as all the other kids, there were some things which made me feel very different. I've always been able to walk short distances without any assistance, but my walking has never been what you'd call steady or straight! My parents were keen to try anything which would help straighten me up and make walking a little bit easier. When I was about seven, my consultant at Sandwell General Hospital recommended that I start wearing splints - basically plastic moulds around my legs and feet which would help me to keep them straight as I walked. We were referred to the Orthopaedic Hospital in Oswestry, Shropshire and, after a consultation, we decided to try the splints. The consultant had to make casts of both my legs. Once they had set, the casts were very carefully cut off so that the moulds could be made. I used to miss quite a bit of school going to these appointments, as a few weeks later we would have to return to the hospital for my new "legs" to be fitted.

As you can imagine, the splints weren't exactly comfortable and I could only wear them with special orthopaedic boots, so they weren't exactly trendy or fashionable either. Whereas most parents took their kids to Clarks for their school shoes, Mum took me to the local hospital! There was never much choice in the boots on offer and I generally had to take what was in stock. I hated being different from the other kids at school and I felt particularly hard done by when the splints began to cause big, painful blisters on my feet.

I used to come home from school, absolutely

desperate to free my feet of the splints. Whenever I got blisters, Mum felt bad for making me wear them and would give me a day or two reprieve from them while the blisters healed. But we both knew that in the long term, the splints would be beneficial and so I continued wearing them for several years and put up with the discomfort.

As I said, my walking could never be described as steady and in the busy playground, it was very common for me to either lose my balance and fall over or be knocked to the ground, albeit innocently, by an over active child. I had many grazed knees in that playground! To eliminate such incidents, I eventually got a walking frame to fly about with. Although a little cumbersome, it gave me a bit more stability and support, so I could roam the playground with my friends.

Although my classmates barely batted an eyelid at these things, there were two lads in the year below who started noticing that I was different. It was in the latter years that they started to bully me. It was nothing physical, but lots of name calling and nasty comments about my walking. Just kids' stuff really - I know now that they just didn't understand why I was different so the easiest thing to do was tease me. I can't even remember when or how it started as I tried my best to ignore it at first, but it started to take its toll on me. Within my classroom, I was no different, but whenever we had to interact with other classes, I began to dread it. The teachers didn't seem to notice, but after a while, Mum realised what was going on and it was like a red rag to a bull! No-one picked on me and got away with it!

Mum went into the school to see the Head and demanded that the culprits be dealt with and she was assured that they would be. Mum left the matter in the school's hands, trusting that they would deal with it. However, despite the school's intervention, the bullies didn't stop,

I was with Mum after school when she spotted one of the "brats" as she called them, outside the school gates. She took him aside and told him in no uncertain terms to leave me alone, otherwise he'd have her to answer to. I don't think the Head fully agreed with Mum's approach and I believe that they had words about it, but regardless, Mum's intervention worked and the bullying stopped immediately.

Chapter 3
True grafters

My parents wanted to have another child soon after me but Mum decided to delay it for a while until I started school. She felt, given the difficulties that I faced, that I needed her undivided attention at least until I was settled at school. I was thrilled at the arrival of my little brother James, in December 1988. Having had three girls, Dad really wanted a son and so James arrived and finally made our family complete. Having two older sisters bossing me about, I was dying to play the big bossy sister myself! I loved helping Mum to look after him. I remember her putting him in my dolls pram and letting me push him up and down the length of our lounge to get him to go to sleep. Collette and Martina were quite a bit older than me and James eventually became my much wished for play mate.

My parents always worked hard to support us - they were and still are true grafters. Dad worked six days a week, sometimes seven, on the buildings. He'd leave the house at six in the morning and not get home until 7 pm. As a little girl, I remember getting up and having breakfast with Dad, before waving him off to work.

Then if he got home before I went to bed, he'd read me a story and say my prayers with me. He wasn't around much, but I knew how hard he worked. Mum also had her hands full looking after all of us, as well as a part-time job in a pub at the weekend.

A few years after James was born, my parents decided to start their own cleaning business; if they were going to work so hard, they might as well reap all of the rewards and so *Houseproud Cleaning* was born. Dad still worked seven days a week but he spent much more time at home. The kitchen table became his office and he'd spend hours writing out staff rotas and doing up the wages. Mum would spend Sunday afternoons phoning all the staff to give them their shifts, then each morning, after she'd taken us to school, she'd be out cleaning with one of the teams. They gave the business all they had and it instilled a good work ethic in us kids. We saw the stress and pitfalls of being self-employed, but we also saw the benefits. Dad always said nobody ever made any money by working for someone else and that to run a successful business you had to 'eat, drink, sleep and take it to the toilet with you!'

Mum and Dad's attitude to hard work meant that we had a brilliant childhood. Each summer we would have a week's holiday and we would either go home to Sligo or have a week at Pontins holiday camp in Southport. Back then, Dad had a silver Cortina and the four of us would squash into the back of it, elbowing and annoying each other while continually moaning to Mum and Dad, 'Are we there yet?' I remember those journeys like they were yesterday! We all felt the relief when we finally rolled up at our destination. We particularly cherished our holidays in Sligo, where we'd stay with Granny in her cottage in Lough Hill.

Granny had twenty-seven grandchildren and she spoilt us all rotten. She had a plaque hanging above the open fire with the instruction, '*If Mother says no, ask Grandma*' and she never let us down! Granny was a fit and active woman, even into her early eighties. She had an old bicycle and she'd regularly cycle the two miles into the village to collect supplies or go to Mass. She was very independent too – that must be where I got it from! Even when we were visiting, she would insist on carrying in buckets of turf for the fire or collecting fresh drinking water from the nearby well. I used to think that water was magic, it tasted that good! My parents would have a few nights out, leaving us in Gran's capable hands. Little did they know that Granny would let us stay up well past bed time, if we kept it a secret! Well, wasn't that what holidays were about? To me, Granny was wonder woman and I absolutely loved staying with her.

Uncle Liam and his family lived across the yard from Granny and he was a wonderful, warm and funny character. He was a farmer and like Dad, he knew the meaning of hard work. I have many fond memories of riding around the fields with Uncle Liam on his quad bike and squealing with delight as Liam revved the bike and took us off like a shot! Those were surely happy holidays.

As well as holidays, my parents always made a big fuss of birthdays and Christmas. Although Dad will happily give Mum all the credit – he's not a big fan of the commercial side of Christmas or of baking birthday cakes! My birthday would always arrive with the pink blossom of the tree in our back garden and I was always blessed with good weather. Just as well because each year, Mum would hire a bouncy castle which would be erected in our back garden for me and my thirty classmates. Our neighbours must have dreaded my birthday. Whatever age I was, Mum would bake a cake in the shape of my age and there'd be presents and cards all over the place.

Mum absolutely loves Christmas and it was always a big occasion in our family. On Christmas Eve, I'd insist on sleeping in my sisters' room – because I was scared that Santa would peer through my curtains and see that I was still awake! I was such an innocent child… As a family, we always had one rule on Christmas morning – nobody was allowed to go downstairs until we were all up and my parents were dressed. I could swear that they deliberately took longer just to keep us all waiting. Eventually, Dad would lead the way downstairs, squint through the living room door and then declare that Santa had forgotten us all this year! Of course, we raced past him to find four big, overflowing sacks of presents.

My parents just wanted me to be like any normal child and despite the endless hospital appointments and the ongoing battle to keep me in mainstream school, I can honestly say that I had an idyllic childhood. Although life wasn't always easy, I was truly blessed with a loving and supportive family who were always there for me.

I was blessed even further with some firm friends who were always there to offer support and encouragement, especially one in particular. Ever since I can remember, Mary Mac was a regular visitor at our home in Jayshaw Avenue. She and my parents have been friends for donkeys' years but it's only recently that I found out how they met. Mary tells me that she knew my aunty Marie first, who lived around the corner from her, and she had asked Marie to recommend someone who could fit some wardrobes. Of course, Marie recommended my Dad and as they say, the rest is history. Mary was always popping in for a natter and a cuppa with Mum and of course, watched me grow up.

She remembers me as a happy, well behaved little girl and I always remember being fond of her. She recalls one day after Mass, when I threw myself into her arms and she began carrying me home, when suddenly she stumbled and fell with me in her arms. She was more concerned about me hitting my head than about any injury she might acquire herself. We both survived the fall without too much fanfare but Mary has never forgotten it!

Something I've never forgotten occurred a few years later when I was about four and visiting Mary. She had a young and playful little dog at the time who took a shine to me. Not being too steady on my feet, this little dog knocked me down on to the kitchen floor and licked me all over! Being so little and unable to get up, the experience left me fearful of dogs for a long time.

As I got older, Mary and I became firm friends and when it came to choosing someone to sponsor me for my Confirmation, there was only one choice and Mary was delighted to support me. Mary is very religious and to this day she takes the responsibility of being my sponsor very seriously and often lectures me about the importance of going to church. She's also responsible for the nick name which has stuck to me for the past sixteen years or so – Tilly Trotter! Mary was reading the book and I can only assume that something about Tilly reminded her of me and from that day to this, I've been known to my family as Tilly, Til or Trotter or whatever version of the nick name comes to mind.

Chapter 4
Does *it* wet the bed?

We're a traditional Irish Catholic family and my faith has always been very important to me. Every Sunday, Mum would dress us in our Sunday best and we'd go to Mass. I was about three when we made our first trip to Lourdes, which is in the South of France. It's famous for the apparitions of Our Lady to St Bernadette in 1858 and many Catholics go on pilgrimage there. The spring water of the grotto is believed to have healing powers, so it's a popular place, particularly for sick pilgrims.

I remember Mum explaining to me that Lourdes was where sick people went and that there were stories over the years of some people being healed. I don't think Mum or Dad ever expected me to be healed but there was always hope, always an attitude of, 'you never know'. For my parents, I think Lourdes just gave them hope and strength, as it later did for me.

Before we continue, I think it's important for me to say that I don't, and never have, considered myself to be 'sick'. That's just the 'speak' of Lourdes, for want of a better phrase! I'm just Aideen and I have a disability. I don't want or need a cure, but nonetheless, Lourdes has always brought me strength and comfort. It has a sense of peace and it's always been a special place for me. I've always said, even if you're not religious, it's a wonderful place to take time out and take stock of life. I'd recommend it to anyone who just wants a peaceful, slow paced break and no, I'm not on commission!

On one of our first pilgrimages, when I was about three or four we were travelling by coach with some of our fellow parishioners. The trip takes about twenty-four hours and we were breaking journey by staying over in a nunnery in Paris. I have very vague memories of this but Mum remembers it vividly. Upon arrival, one of the nuns took one look at me and without blinking, asked Mum, 'Does *IT* wet the bed?'

Needless to say, Mum was absolutely furious. She didn't care that this was a Nun – she had no right to insult me in the way she had and Mum wasn't about to hold back! She told her in no uncertain terms that I was NOT an 'it', my name was Aideen and no, I did *not* wet the bed! Mum could hardly believe the audacity in those five words. The cheeky side of me thinks it's a shame that I didn't wet the bed that night!

Nonetheless, Mum and I continued to make many trips to Lourdes over the years. Unfortunately, as it was quite expensive we could never make the trip as a whole family, but sometimes Dad came with us and on other occasions, Collette and Martina took turns to join us. I remember one particular trip when Collette was with us. The hotel had been booked through the parish and when we arrived it was an absolute hovel; Mum refused to stay in it. I remember the three of us trailing around Lourdes, Mum pushing me and Collette trying to carry the luggage, looking for an alternative hotel. It reminds me of Mary and Joseph and the 'no room at the inn' story!

When I was about seven, we were approached by one of the parish priests about an opportunity to make a picture book about my visits. The book would be published by Penguin and would be used in schools and churches to teach other children about Lourdes. It was to be my first claim to fame and I was so excited when the photographer arrived to take the pictures. The book would be entitled 'My Book' and it had a series of pictures of me with various symbols of Lourdes – the holy water, rosary beads etc. Dad still has a copy of the book and it's funny to look back on what a holy, awfully serious child I appeared to be!

When I was a little older, I had the opportunity to go to Lourdes with a youth group and with a support worker. This was my first time to be away from the family and it gave my parents a break and an opportunity to spend some time with Collette, Martina and James. When my support worker phoned Mum each evening, I think she was a little upset to learn that I was having a great time and didn't have time to talk to her. Sorry about that Mum!

It was during my secondary education that I became involved with Birmingham's Catholic Handicapped Fellowship. The group was run by the family of one of my classmates and they invited me to join the group. Each Saturday the group celebrated Mass, which was always followed by a social gathering and a natter. My classmate Mark and his Dad used to pick me up in their mini-bus, which we called the 'Smiley Bus' and then drop me home later in the evening. It was a good way of me getting out and meeting people and I began to look forward to Saturdays.

Each year, the group went to Lourdes for a week and I was in my first year of college when I decided to join their pilgrimage. One of my college friends had suddenly passed away and it had been quite a shock for me. Death had fortunately not been that close to me before and I was finding it quite difficult to deal with. I returned home for half-term and rang Mark to tell him that I was back. He said they were leaving for Lourdes in the morning and he happened to mention that someone had pulled out of the trip at the last minute.

After the grief and sadness of the previous few

weeks, I knew that I needed a break, so after talking Mum round, I packed my case and early the next morning, I was on a coach headed for my special place. As always, the trip brought me a lot of peace and helped me to come to terms with what had happened at college. Mark had said that there would be someone my own age who would support me for the week. We took the ferry to Calais and then travelled overnight by train down to Lourdes. It was a long, tiring trip but it was great fun. Although the week was quite rightly filled with various Masses, services and quiet time, there was also plenty of play time, normally in the various pubs or back at the hotel bar each night!

I was so glad that I'd made the decision to go and that was cemented further when I met Ian. He was travelling with another pilgrimage and we joined his group during one of the evening candlelit processions. Ian has three children of his own, all in and around my age. He instantly took me under his wing and after returning from Lourdes, we became solid friends. He lived locally to the college where I was studying in Coventry and he'd pop over on his motorbike to visit me. I am so thankful that I went that year – it brought me so much peace and I gained much more than I ever thought possible.

I enjoyed those trips immensely, but as I got older and more independent, I found being in a group all week and doing everything together a little suffocating. On one trip, I managed to bring my electric wheelchair, in the hope of getting some time alone. However, the pilgrimage leaders frowned upon this and I got frustrated. I was after all by now an adult and I was capable of living independently. I loved Lourdes and I craved time on my own, just to soak it all in and take time out, as they say. That was difficult to do and so unfortunately, it's now been over five years since I last went.

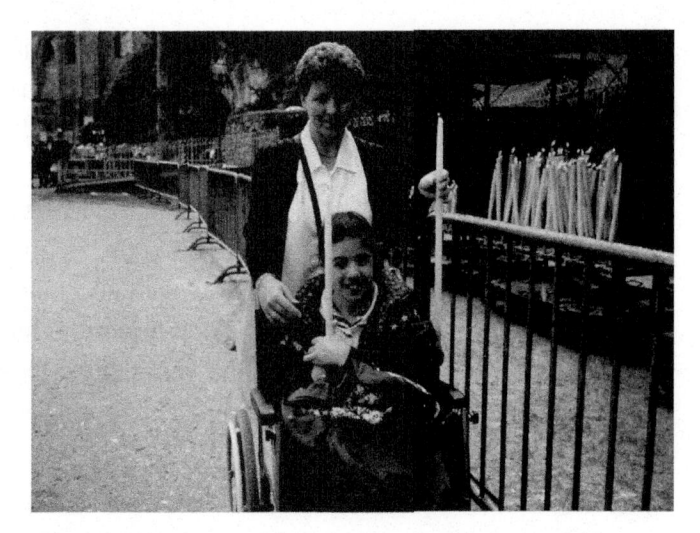

Mum and I made many trips to Lourdes over the years and it became my special place.

Chapter 5
If at first you don't succeed...

As I've said, in my parents' eyes, I was no different to any other child and they didn't want me to be treated differently just because I had cerebral palsy. They wanted me to achieve as much as possible and gave me every opportunity to do so. If I wanted to try something, Mum and Dad supported me to have a go, even though they must have known some things would prove too difficult for me.

Firstly, there was the Irish Dancing. Collette and Martina went to classes every Saturday morning and Mum took me along to watch. I was desperate to do it too, so Mum asked if I could join the junior group. Mum knew that I could barely walk, let alone do Irish Dancing, but me being me, I had to at least try before I'd accept that dancing wasn't for me! Collette and Martina on the other hand, excelled at Irish Dancing and competed in loads of competitions, including the World Championships in which Martina won second place. I used to go along and watch them get dressed up and although I really wished I could do it as well, I enjoyed watching and cheering them on.

Then there was swimming. Every class in the school went swimming once a week, but there was one problem and Mum clashed with the Head again. Even though I had one-to-one support provided by my nursery nurse, the Head was extremely concerned about my safety in the water and didn't want to put this huge responsibility on the nurse. But Mum wasn't prepared to let me miss out, so she met us at the swimming pool, helped me get ready then sat by the pool to watch. We had an excellent swimming instructor and seeing my apprehension and nervousness in the water, he gave me a lane all to myself so that I could concentrate without being knocked by the other kids. It took lots of time, practice and encouragement, but eventually I could swim a significant distance without any support or floats. It was a huge achievement for me, one which even I did not think possible at the beginning. But it was only made possible by Mum's compromise with the Head and the determined instructor who refused to give up on me. I was even able to take part in the lifeguard challenge during Year Six, which involved being able to swim while fully clothed. I was so proud of my achievements that, during the summer holidays, Mum enrolled me on a swimming programme so that I could continue to practice.

Dad also encouraged physical activity and although I didn't have the balance to ride a traditional bike, that didn't deter me. Mum and Dad brought me a tricycle, a huge blue thing it was and most weekends, Dad and I would head up to our local park so that I could race around on it. Although it was different to what the other kids had, I really didn't care. I felt just like any other kid as I built up speed and whizzed around the park. It was quite hilly though, so Dad had a tough time helping me up hills and then holding me back as I went flying over the other side! I thought it was great fun, but I'm sure it was exhausting for him!

Thanks to my parents' 'can do' philosophy, there was very little that I wouldn't try, and my sense of adventure even extended to horse riding. My best friend at school, Lynsey, absolutely loved animals and had started riding lessons. Like most kids, I was keen to be just like my friends and have everything they had. So I begged Mum for riding lessons and eventually she booked a lesson as a treat for my birthday. But never seeing myself as any different, I hadn't really thought this through: I soon realised that I didn't have the balance to ride a horse. I circled the paddock with someone supporting me and I really enjoyed it, but I knew that I'd never be able to ride independently. Mum probably knew that in the first place, but I'm grateful that she and Dad always gave me the opportunity to at least try things and realise my limitations for myself, even if on occasions they were hard to accept.

As I grew older and even more head strong and determined, it often took me even longer to accept defeat. When I started at Hereward College at the age of sixteen, I found out that if you were registered disabled, you were allowed to start learning to drive early (at the age of 16, rather than 17). There was a specialist instructor who had an adapted car and taught a lot of the students at the college. My mind was already made up: I was going to learn to drive.

The instructor, John, first arranged an assessment which would test my ability to control a vehicle and also check the speed of my reactions. If I passed the assessment, I'd be able to apply for a provisional driving licence and start my lessons. Within a few weeks, he took me out for my first lesson and I absolutely loved it! I used hand controls to drive as the assessment had concluded that my reactions with my feet weren't fast enough but my hand reactions were much quicker. I began having regular lessons and surprisingly, I wasn't a bad driver! It took some time to build my confidence, but once I had it I felt really in control and I loved my lessons with John. In time, he felt I was ready to take my test and I agreed: that was the point where I came unstuck.

I could drive confidently with John sitting beside me. But the moment the test instructor took his place, nerves took over and my confidence disappeared. I kept making silly mistakes and as the test progressed,

I knew that I'd failed. I never expected to pass my test first time but nor did I expect to take it seven times. Yes, you read that correctly. SEVEN TIMES!

I'd love to say that it was seventh time lucky, but it wasn't. By this point, my time at Hereward was coming to an end and I was moving on to pastures new. It would be difficult to find another specialist driving instructor and to be honest, after seven attempts, I was feeling a little deflated. I didn't necessarily *need* to drive. It was just something that I really wanted to prove that I could to, both to myself and everyone else. The freedom and independence of being able to drive would have been great, but I felt it was time to accept that it was a dream I might not be able to achieve. That was difficult as I never accept failure easily! But I decided to take a break from driving, with the full intention of going back to it at some point. As often happens, life takes over and I never resumed my lessons, but I was glad that I'd had the opportunity to at least *try*.

But that wasn't the only new opportunity that Hereward College presented me with. During my final year, the college were planning a trip to an outdoor adventure centre, The Calvert Trust, in the Lake District and it was specifically designed for disabled people. There was absolutely no way that I was missing out on it and as places were limited, I put my name down straight away. I would have to raise the cost of the trip through sponsorship, so I decided to do a 24 hour awake-a-thon. As my fellow students slept, I managed to stay awake all night, reading and watching TV. Having raised the money for my trip, I couldn't wait until my 19th birthday - the day we were heading off on our adventure.

I wasn't disappointed! I had a go at everything that the centre had to offer including sailing, archery and indoor rock climbing. Having always been a dare devil, I loved every minute of it and couldn't get enough of it. By the end of the week, I really didn't want to leave. The experience really opened even my eyes to the support which is available for disabled people and I was able to do things that I'd never even dreamt of. The staff at the centre were truly amazing and made anything possible. Who'd have thought that I'd ever be capable of rock climbing?

Chapter 6
A local celebrity

When I was about eight years old, Mum and Dad were told about a new type of 'therapy' called Conductive Education (CE) which could potentially make a big difference to me. I was having regular physiotherapy at the local hospital, but CE had been developed specifically for children with CP and it was a very intense form of treatment. It was devised by Professor Andras Peto, who came from Hungary and is a learning system specifically for individuals with motor disorders. The treatment was now available in the UK and there was a Peto Centre in London

My parents had heard how good CE was and how much it could benefit me. Don't get me wrong, it isn't a cure – cerebral palsy can't be reversed, but CE can do a lot to help the individual to control their movements. It's like training the brain to think more carefully about the movements the body is making and through practice, make the brain react differently. Eventually, the movements require less thought and become more naturally controlled.

My parents decided that it was worth a try and so Mum and I set off to the Peto Centre. However, the programme wasn't cheap and in order to have any long lasting effects, I would need to keep returning to London whenever possible. This was to put a substantial financial strain on Mum and Dad.

As soon as the local community found out about the programme and its financial implications, we were blown away by their generosity. People started organising fundraising events in my name to contribute towards the cost of sending me to London. Some people organised sponsored walks, others planned Irish Dance nights. There were activities going on all over the place, all to support me. I was absolutely amazed at how much people cared and I remember feeling a little bit like a local celebrity! Everyone seemed to know about me and the treatment and the support was overwhelming.

We were particularly touched by one of my sister's friends, Mark. He had just turned eighteen and had received a few hundred pounds as a birthday present. He came round to see me and donated all the money to my 'fund'. Even at my young age, I was overwhelmed by his kindness and I hope he knows how grateful I am to him, even today. It was kind enough of people to raise money for me, but to donate his own money was particularly touching and I've never forgotten it. Thanks Mark!

The kindness of the local community gave me a feeling of responsibility and determination – I was so grateful that I committed myself to working as hard as I could during the programme. So Mum and I spent many of my half-term breaks down in London. We'd stay at the Peto Centre and each day at 9 am, Mum would take me down to the programme leaders and the hard work would begin.

The day was pretty gruelling and would consist of several sessions – some lying down, some sitting, standing and walking, as well as some art work which was designed to assist hand and eye coordination. There was a lot of repetition in the activities as it was designed to train the brain and make it remember how to control the movements. Even during meal times, the instructors would ensure that we were sitting and using the cutlery correctly. There was no let up and the days were really tiring. It was like I had swapped one school for another, but I didn't resent the loss of my holidays. I knew the programme had the potential to make a huge difference to me and so many people had donated money to make it possible. I felt a huge responsibility to work as hard as I could so that I'd benefit as much as possible from the programme and people would hopefully be able to see the difference it had made.

Although the programme was hard work and I was

often exhausted, the evenings were fun. During one of the first visits to London, we met Jenny and Chris. Chris is slightly younger than me and also has CP. His mum Jenny has an Irish background, so she and Mum hit it off straight away. So while Chris and I were working hard, Mum and Jenny kept each other company. There were many shopping trips too!

The four of us would eat together in the shared accommodation and then pass the evenings playing cards and watching television. I dare say Mum and Jenny shared a few drinks after we'd been put to bed too! At least once during the week, the four of us would go to Oxford and Regent street and as a treat for working so hard, we'd go to the big toy shop Hamleys. As a child, I can't tell you how big that place seems! It's a kid's idea of Heaven!

But on one particular evening, Mum had an extra special treat in store. We were going to the theatre to see 'Joseph and his Amazing Technicolor Dreamcoat', starring Jason Donovan. It was the highlight of my week, especially when Mum managed to arrange for me to meet Jason after the show. To say I was star struck is a bit of an understatement! I'd grown up watching this guy on Neighbours and now, I was talking to him and having my photo taken with him! It made all the hard work worth it and was my second claim to fame.

The programme had a noticeable effect on my CP and for weeks after each programme, people commented on how much my balance and general coordination had improved. I noticed it too, I felt straighter and much more in control of my movements. So for the next few years, Mum and I went to London whenever possible and we even spent 3 weeks of one summer break in the Peto Centre in Sheffield. I think they used to take over Sheffield University during the summer holidays. Although I still worked as hard as I could, Sheffield wasn't half as much fun as London and it was further from home, so I only remember going there for one programme.

As I approached starting secondary school, it wasn't practical to continue with the programme and it tended to have better results with younger children, so eventually we stopped going. We kept in touch with Jenny and Chris and got to know each other's families. We are still firm friends today and Jenny would never forgive me if I didn't tell you all a secret. All those years ago, Jenny encouraged me to write a book and said if I did, I'd have to give her a mention. So there it is – I've fulfilled a 20 year old promise and I have Jenny to thank that this has been published!

Chapter 7
Speaking up for myself

If there's one thing that really used to bug Mum and me, it was when people used to just assume that I didn't have a brain and they would talk to her rather than me, as if I wasn't even there. Questions such as, 'Aww, what's her name?' or, 'Would she like a drink?' would frustrate and upset me and drive Mum mad. She always made a point of never answering for me – if anyone wanted such information, they could talk to me directly. After all, I did have a brain and always had plenty to say for myself! That was until I was ten and I realised how much I took that for granted.

I was in Year Six at school and having made it this far against all odds, it was a year of uncertainty and change. In a few months' time, I was going to be moving on to secondary school. But once again, despite everything I had achieved, the powers that be had doubts about how I would cope in an entirely different environment which would present a new set of challenges. For one, I wouldn't be based in just one classroom – I would have to move around for each of my classes. Secondly, all the nearest secondary schools were a drive away and unlike my friends, I'd be unable to get the bus to school and would need the Local Education Authority (LEA) to fund my transport by taxi. I would still need a full-time assistant and as the school had so many stairs, I'd have to walk from class to class which would put a physical strain on us both. As well as being physically exhausted, there would be a lot more homework to concentrate on each evening. It was going to be a big change for me and I think everyone, including myself to some degree, worried that I may not cope. However, I'd got this far and there was no way on earth I was giving up now. As far as I was concerned, I was going to secondary school with my friends and that was that! Mum and Dad's stubbornness regarding my mainstream education had rubbed off on me. Eventually, it was agreed that I would be going to the same school as most of my friends and that support would be put in place. It seemed that my future Headmaster would be very supportive!

However, some of my peers were doubtful that I would overcome the challenges and I remember one particular break-time in the playground talking about the impending changes with two of my 'friends'. They rather bluntly informed me that they didn't see me lasting more than a week in our new secondary school. Kids tend not to be very tactful and I remember being hurt and angered that even my so-called friends doubted me, but looking back, they were 11 year old kids who were probably only repeating the comments of their parents. But it made me more determined that not only would I last more than a week, I'd last right through to the completion of my GCSEs and even beyond that, to my A-levels.

It was during this final turbulent year at primary school that I went on my first 'mainstream' Guide Camp. It was only a weekend so Mum agreed that I could go. I looked forward to the trip for weeks and loved the idea of camping with my friends, talking half the night and fooling around. I took my manual wheelchair with me and as I was unable to move myself very far, Mum and I were assured that the Guide Leaders would manage to push me around the field.

However, when we arrived at the camp site it became evident that it would not be so easy for me to get around – as you might expect, the field we were camping in wasn't very even and was very muddy, which made it difficult to push the wheelchair across it. The Guide Leaders suggested I try walking a little bit – something which I embraced because it made me feel more like the other girls, although obviously I wasn't as quick…

We had great fun putting up tents, orienteering and all the other typical guide camp activities. But I wasn't used to so much physical activity and I was beginning to tire: all the walking, combined with very little sleep was taking it out of me and I really needed my wheelchair again. At one point, I remember asking for it because I knew I was physically exhausted but nobody brought it to me. By the time we boarded the coach on Sunday afternoon to go home, I had had enough and I slept all the way back.

Getting off the coach, I was met by Mum and I tried to greet her and tell her about my trip. I realised my jaw was stiff. I couldn't control my mouth to form the words that were in my head. I was so tired, I could barely speak! Mum was told about all the walking I'd done and took me home for a good night's sleep. I was convinced I'd wake up the next day, full of beans. Instead, this was the start of an absolute nightmare which saw me sink into myself and feel more isolated than I'd ever been before.

The next day, my speech was no better. It was as if my jaw was locked. Each time I tried to speak, I was battling to get free, but I just couldn't; the words were in my head, but my mouth just couldn't form them. It was scary: one day, everyone could understand me perfectly and the next, even those closest to me could barely understand a word. What was going on? Why didn't anyone get it? I felt as if I was locked in my own little world and no matter how hard I tried, I couldn't escape.

Mum soon realised this was more serious than me just being tired. When things didn't improve, she took me to the doctors to try and find some answers. Everyone wondered whether my impending move to a new school and all the uncertainty was worrying me and whether all my anxiety had manifested itself in this physical problem. I had concerns about my new school, but I had not been that anxious. If anything, I was more anxious now. If even my family couldn't understand me, how could I expect new friends and teachers to get what I was saying? But of course, it was impossible to explain any of this.

It was particularly hard for Mum and Dad. They had always understood every word I was saying and now even they could barely communicate with me. The frustration of having to repeat everything over and over again and still not be understood, angered and upset me. I wasn't angry at people for not understanding, but at myself, for being unable to make people understand. What was wrong with me? Why couldn't I just speak clearly again? Sometimes I decided it wasn't worth the effort and just said, 'It doesn't matter'. It wasn't like me at all to just give up and I hated myself for it, but I became so frustrated, I just didn't know what else to do. It was exhausting, trying to form the words over and over again, battling against this 'lock' that had plunged me into this frustrated state.

But Mum was reluctant to let me give up and would

encourage me to say things again but slower. I remember one evening walking into the kitchen to ask her for a drink. I must have asked her five or six times and I couldn't even get this simple sentence across – I don't know which one of us was more frustrated. In the end I walked off to get a piece of paper and used this to tell her what I wanted. It was a last resort and one of the only times in my life when I began giving up, taking the easy route.

This went on for months and nobody could understand or explain it, least of all me. I was sent for speech therapy and blood tests, but nothing seemed to provide the answers. Eventually, my GP decided to send me for an MRI Scan – a prospect which terrified me. Mum took me to the hospital and my fear meant the nurses had a hard time getting the scan because my head kept shaking. Whenever they tried to move me into the scanner I panicked and my positioning was wrong again. This was the first time that I realised I was claustrophobic. Both Mum and the nurses were getting quite frustrated, but I just couldn't help it – the thought of being trapped in a narrow tunnel, which moved and made strange noises, sent me loopy! It was no use, so in the end they decided to do the scan while I was under general anaesthetic. Mum joked that when they finally did the scan, they would discover my brain was missing – cheers Mum!

I would love to say that the scan revealed the cause

of my severe speech deterioration and that everything was explained and put right. The truth is, the scan revealed that I did in fact have a brain and that everything was as would be expected. The doctors, Mum, Dad and I were all baffled – nobody could explain why my speech had gone downhill so quickly, so nobody knew how to put it right. I've normally found CP to be quite predictable and I know where I stand with it, but on this occasion it definitely took us all by surprise. As I've said, no two people with CP are the same, it affects people in different ways and so the doctors had no similar cases to compare. It was certainly one of the most difficult periods I've had to deal with.

Although over time and to everyone's relief, my speech did improve, even now I still have brief spells when my jaw locks and I feel like it's happening all over again. But it generally only happens when I'm either really tired, particularly stressed or both. I find it happens more if I'm talking to someone I don't know and I get a little anxious about them being able to understand me, which is ironic! These days, my husband Dean is very good at picking up when my jaw is tense and reminds me to count to ten. This usually gives me time to relax and my speech returns to 'normal' – whatever that is! So perhaps in hindsight, the incident when I was ten was due to stress and I've just learnt to manage it, who knows? I don't think we'll ever know.

As my final year at primary school came to a close and I prepared for starting my new school, my speech began to stabilise again and it only affected me when I got tired or stressed. A new chapter approached, I was anxious, but also excited and driven by determination. My last day at Holy Name RC Primary School was a triumph for us all, though probably more of a relief to my Headmistress! There were lots of tears as I said goodbye to one chapter of my life and prepared to embrace another.

Chapter 8

Head down and mouth shut

Mum and Dad had fought for eight long years to keep me in mainstream education and now here I was, about to start a new school – St Francis of Assisi in Aldridge, Walsall. So many people had doubted I'd get this far, it felt like a huge achievement and it proved Mum and Dad had been right to fight for my place in the school. Now I had to prove my own peers wrong – I had to survive the additional challenges of a mainstream secondary school for much longer than a week.

For the past four years, I'd been supported by a lovely Polish lady and we worked well together. I really liked her and I knew that she really wanted to move with me to St. Francis. But once again, the authorities and the Head had different ideas and after much confusion, my new support worker for secondary school, Mrs Clarke, was appointed. I don't think she will mind me saying that I was a little apprehensive at first. I didn't understand why my current nursery nurse couldn't move to my new school with me and we were both quite upset at the decision. But nonetheless, Mrs

Clarke was introduced to me during my final weeks at Holy Name and despite my previous upset, we seemed to get on well.

St Francis was a big school, with seven classes in each year group plus a Sixth Form. It was out in the country really, well as country as you can get in the West Midlands! The school was well spread out, with a huge playing field and it accommodated almost a thousand pupils. Some might question why my parents wanted me to go to a school that wasn't wheelchair accessible and would be physically exhausting for me. But the school had the best reputation of any Catholic secondary school in our area and the majority of my friends were going there. Also, Mum and Dad didn't want me being in a wheelchair all day, they have always encouraged me to have as much mobility as possible and I've embraced that. Just like before, they knew with the right support it was well within my capabilities to thrive at St. Francis.

However, we all knew that this was going to be a big change! But this time, I had the full support of my Headmaster and the school did everything possible to help me. The seven classes of each year group were labelled F-R-A-N-C-I-S and each group represented a different level of ability – with F being the highest. I was assessed as being in group N – slap bang in the middle and although it meant being in a different class to many of my primary school friends, I was happy. As I always had, I excelled at English and as soon as this was realised, I moved up a few sets for English and continued to enjoy it.

Mrs Clarke and I settled in well and we became quite a team. I was given a portable word processor to complete all my written work and as soon as I printed out my work, Mrs Clarke would cut it to size and stick it in my exercise books. We had a good system going and I never got marked down for bad handwriting! As I'd expected, St Francis was physically hard work for both of us. My lessons were spread out all over the place and Mrs Clarke carried my school bag and word processor, as well as giving me support as I walked. Whenever we could, we left classes 5 minutes early just so we could get to the next lesson on time. Sometimes, I'd have to climb up several flights of stairs to get to our classroom and would often be exhausted after school, but I soon got used to my new environment and routine.

Mrs Clarke has a son just 3 days older than me. He had started at another local secondary school at the same time and sitting in on my lessons was no doubt useful to her in following her son's school work. She often said that she was learning just as much as me, particularly when it came to the French lessons! Mrs Clarke was invaluable and I was incredibly lucky to have her. With her constant support, I was able to participate in everything my peers did, including art and woodwork, as well as cookery and PE.

Whenever my class were doing something really physically challenging like cross country running, Mrs Clarke would devise a one-to-one session for me with exercises to help build up my muscle strength and coordination. She always made sure time was put to the best use and kept me focused, even when I really didn't want to be! I didn't always appreciate the things she did, but now I am so extremely grateful for the time and effort she put into supporting me.

Just like I had at Holy Name, I was thriving at St Francis and I was really enjoying the new challenges that being there presented. Being a bit older and wiser, my sisters had given me a pep-talk about the pitfalls of secondary school and I thought that I was prepared for the inevitable bullies. It started quite subtly. The occasional evil eye, the odd comment. If anyone had ever asked me to define a bully, I'd probably have described someone who used verbal and physical abuse to intimidate their chosen victim. That's why this particular bully persisted for so long. It sounds stupid now, but initially I didn't realise that I was being bullied and I didn't consider myself a victim. She was very manipulative and the things she did, if noticed, couldn't immediately be construed as bullying. But she was a tall, domineering girl, her demeanour was threatening and I didn't fancy my chances if she tried anything physical.

On one occasion, she was sitting behind me in a music lesson and began kicking the back of my chair. I tried to just ignore it because when I turned around, she gave me a nasty, threatening look as if to say, 'Yeah, what are you going to do about it?' It was really difficult to concentrate and Mrs Clarke noticed my distraction, but whenever Mrs Clarke turned around she smiled sweetly as if she wasn't doing anything. Butter wouldn't melt, yeah right!

Everyone in the school knew she was a trouble maker, but unfortunately, as these people often are, she was fairly popular and standing up to someone like that is difficult.

The little incidents went on for a while. I used to dread bumping into her in the toilets or at lunch time as she became a little braver and the abuse became more verbal. One lunch time, she was nearby as I asked my best friend to put something in the bin for me, purely because she was closer to it. A perfectly reasonable request, but she overheard and piped up to my friend, telling her to make me do it myself. On another occasion, she was chosen to work with me in a PE lesson and again, she was as nice as pie when Mrs Clarke was watching, but as soon as her back was turned, she'd turn on me, making me feel intimidated with her looks and snide comments. I know it doesn't sound much and that's why I couldn't tell anyone. It was the way she looked at me as she said things, it made me feel threatened and vulnerable.

But how pathetic would it sound to say 'She's giving me nasty looks', or 'She's telling my friends not to help me', or 'She keeps kicking my chair.' Sounds so petty and stupid, doesn't it? I couldn't prove that I was being bullied, but with all the incidents adding up and her general reputation as a trouble maker, I was scared of her and of what she might be building up to. So for months, I kept my head down and my mouth shut. I felt that nobody would believe I was being bullied.

It all came to a head one Valentine's Day when we were in Year 8. I'd decided to be brave and put a message in the school magazine for the lad I'd fancied since primary school. The only problem was, the girl who had been picking on me was collating all the messages. I plucked up the courage to give her the message and unusually, she was as nice as pie; I should have known better than to trust her. When my message was printed, it was signed with her name! I was upset as it had taken a lot for me to write the message and now she had taken the credit. It was petty and stupid, but it was another little dig that she knew would upset me. But again, how could I report it? I would be told to ignore her, but trying to do that was becoming increasingly difficult. She always seemed to be there, bugging and annoying me, goading me for a reaction, taking pleasure from seeing me upset. She knew she had the upper hand and that I was too scared to take control.

That weekend, out of the blue, she turned up at my local youth club. It was the one place I hadn't expected to see her, the one place I thought I could relax as she lived in a different area. After the Valentine's incident, it was all too much. I can't remember exactly what happened, but I think she must have started taunting me about the Valentine's thing and I finally broke down in tears in front of everyone. I'd finally had enough and I think I wanted people to know what had been going on. It came out in front of everyone, including the lad that I'd fancied, what she'd done. I think it was apparent to all from my reaction to her that night that there was a much bigger issue.

This wasn't about a silly, childish Valentines message; I couldn't care less about that now. This was months of anguish, frustration and fear coming to a head. I'd finally had enough and I think I suddenly realised how much stress and pain she had caused me. After months of keeping things to myself and hoping against hope that she would get bored, everything was now out in the open and my closest friends began to realise the pressure that I'd been under. It was a relief, but I now had to take control and make it stop.

That night, I finally told Mum what had been going on. I think she was surprised that I'd held it in this long, but I still felt silly: this girl hadn't physically hurt me, but I realise now she was psychologically wearing me down until I snapped. It didn't matter that it was nothing specific and that I couldn't put my finger on it. That's almost what made it worse, she knew there wasn't any proof of what she was doing, so I wouldn't say anything. But she was bullying me and I knew now that it had to stop.

Mum encouraged me to talk to Mrs Clarke, who knew what this girl was like. Even though Mrs Clarke was with me most of the time, she had managed to conceal most of it from her. Mrs Clarke asked me to start noting down whenever she did anything so that we could then report her. But before I could gather any evidence and much to my huge relief, she managed to get herself expelled. I don't think it was because of me, but that probably didn't help her.

I've learnt a lot since then and have realised that bullying comes in lots of different forms. The majority of bullying isn't physical, but it still hurts just as much. People can appear to be as nice as pie to your face, but that doesn't mean there isn't anything going on under the surface. These days, I'm much more confident and feisty, but back then I didn't have the experience to realise when the line had been crossed.

I wish I'd had the confidence just to talk to someone about what was going on, but I was afraid people would think that I was being silly. I realise now that nobody would have thought that and I would urge anyone who is being bullied just to talk to someone. From then on, nobody bothered me and I got on with achieving my goal – getting to and passing my GCSEs.

Chapter 9
Summer of '97

Although I had a good group of friends at school, I never quite felt fully included. This wasn't helped by the fact that the Headteacher had recommended that I spend my breaks and lunchtimes in the school canteen, rather than in the outdoor areas where I could take a fall without Mrs Clarke being there to support me. While I understood and respected this decision, it meant that I couldn't mix with the others and my circle of friends was limited to the couple who were allowed to stay with me in the canteen. These were my two best friends from Holy Name, Lynsey and Linzi. Although I knew they didn't mind staying in with me, I sometimes felt guilty. At weekends, Lynsey would often walk up to my house and take me out locally. We'd look around the shops and then she would take me home again. I was incredibly grateful to her for those little shopping trips, but quite often I felt like a burden. I longed to be like any other teenager and be able to go out when it pleased me, rather than rely on my family and friends to take me out.

All that changed and I got my wish in the summer of

1997 when I was twelve. My uncle Gerald, who is also my Godfather, asked me to go and stay with him in Dublin during the summer holidays. My cousin Gemma is only six months older than me so it would be a great opportunity to spend some time with her. Mum was a little apprehensive as she put me on my first solo flight to Dublin. But needless to say, I was so excited I just couldn't wait to get going. The flight attendants looked after me well and Gerald was there to meet me when I landed.

I was soon to realise that life in Dublin was a lot different to life in Birmingham and a lot more fun! I'd barely unpacked my case before Gemma was taking me to hang out with her friends, who I soon referred to as 'the gang'! Brian, Stacey, Amy, Sinead, Laura, Eimear and Jessica welcomed me with open arms and I soon became one of them. I was only 'home' for a week but it was jam packed with fun! The gang took turns pushing me around in my wheelchair, having great fun doing wheelies with me! We went bowling and swimming, we hung out on *The Green* for hours on end, gossiping and fooling around. For the first time ever, I felt like I belonged. Nobody cared or even noticed that I was different and that was good. I was never left out of anything and was just like any other normal teenager. Our favourite pastime was swimming, but only because most of us fancied the life guard who was often on duty! We'd compete for his attention and then talk about nothing else all the way home! Occasionally, we'd all pile into the back of Gerard's van and he'd take us to the coast – usually a small seaside town called Bray, not far from Dublin. In the back of that van and fooling around in the sea and on the beach we'd have great *craic*, which is an Irish expression meaning to have fun and banter!

From then on, my summer trips to Dublin became a regular occurrence and I looked forward to that one week all year, while desperately missing my new friends. Letters went back and forth, over the Irish Sea and I loved arriving home from school to find my name scrawled across an envelope with an Irish post mark! During my second summer trip, I became involved with the local summer Palmerstown Youth Group. They organised trips and activities throughout the summer holidays and allowed me to take part. One year, they had a disco to mark the end of the summer programme and I was awarded a trophy for taking part. We all danced the night away and I was in my element! Mum and Dad never let me outside the front door in Birmingham, for fear of what might happen or who might be hanging around. In contrast, my uncle Gerry hardly knew I was there, I was that occupied, but he knew that I was safe and it was a breath of fresh air having so much freedom.

The gang became a huge part of my teenage years and I looked forward to my trips with great excitement. We all kept in touch in between my trips. The girls all knew and teased me about my soft spot for Brian too! There was a song out at the time by Alanis Morissette called '*Head over Feet*'. We all loved it and the lyrics went, '*You treat me like I'm a princess*' and every time it came on, the girls used to sing it at me - replacing the 'you' for 'he' and giving a wink! Brian did treat me like a princess, but he was the first friend I'd ever had that I didn't feel like a burden on.

He called for me whenever he could, taking me for walks and when I returned to Birmingham, writing to me and phoning whenever we were allowed to. I'll never forget the first letter Brian sent to me, saying he missed me. He'd signed it with 'love you' and I accidentally let Mum read it! Needless to say, the teasing went on for days and Mum already had me married off!

When we were fourteen, we arranged for Brian to come and visit me for a weekend in Birmingham. As always, it was packed full of fun and we got on well. Brian is what I'd call a 'cheeky chappie' and Mum and Dad took to him immediately. I think they were pleased I'd found a true, genuine friend and from then on Mum and Dad always welcomed him into our home and invited him to family events. Although they knew he was as mad as a hatter, they also knew that he'd look after me well. As we grew older and my parents moved back to Sligo, Brian would come and visit me whenever I was at home. He'd take me out on the town and it was the only time I'd get away with staying out until 4am!! We'd drink until the sun came up and the bars threw us out! Then Brian would push me around the town, fooling around, until I eventually managed to bundle us both into a taxi heading for our house in Calry!

On one of Brian's visits to Sligo, it was a beautiful sunny day and Mum agreed to drive us out to Rosses Point – a seaside town just ten minutes from my parents' home in Calry. It's one of my favourite places and whenever I'm home, Dad takes me out there to watch the sunset. It's absolutely beautiful and I always feel at peace there, no matter what's happening.

On this occasion, we took our Labrador, Sandy, for a run around on the beach. Mum took care of Sandy, while Brian took me down onto the beach in my manual wheelchair. Despite the sand being a bit wet, we had a good walk, but I knew it was hard work on Brian pushing me across the sand. We decided to head back to the car, which unfortunately meant climbing back up a steep, sandy hill back to the car park.

But Brian was puffed out and he'd had enough. All of a sudden, he'd turfed me out of the wheelchair and began pushing it up the hill. I was laughing so hard as I began stumbling up the hill, all the while thinking that Brian would be waiting for me with the chair when I finally reached the top. But as I huffed and puffed up the hill, I saw Brian up ahead getting into the wheelchair and starting to wheel himself away across the car park. Mum was somewhere behind me and we were both laughing and yelling at him to stop being an eejit! But Brian was getting up quite a speed and then bang! He managed to topple himself backwards and now, there he was, legs dangling in the air, unable to move! Worse still, two old ladies were running towards the eejit to rescue him. Through our tears of laughter, Mum and I tried to reassure them that he was only messing around and wasn't worthy of their concern! Once I finally got back into the wheelchair, I was shattered but I think the three of us laughed all the way back home, remembering the look of horror on those ladies' faces!

Brian was the apple of my eye for a long time and he knew it! But the truth was, he was and remains one of my best friends. Even though our lives are busy and we may not speak that often, I know he'll always be my best friend. Like Mum and Dad, he has always believed in me and offered encouragement and support, even when I doubted myself. His friendship and support was to see me through many trying times.

Chapter 10
Another battle

I was in Year 10, when once again Mrs Clarke went above and beyond what was expected of her. My Mum had gone to Ireland for the weekend as my Nan had had a heart attack and was in hospital. Mum wasn't sure if she would pull through, so she took the first available flight to be with her in Dublin. Dad was still working seven days a week, keeping the cleaning business going which left my eldest sister, Collette, with responsibility for getting James and I ready for school.

I woke up on the Monday morning with a bad stomach ache. I always loved school and it took a lot to keep me away. Dad and Collette had to go to work so I went to school as normal. But as the day wore on, I was in agony and could barely walk. I had never known pain like it and I was scared. Mrs Clarke took me to the school sick bay, by which time I was screaming and crying with pain and the school called Collette to collect me. I think she felt bad for sending me to school, but it wasn't her fault, the pain hadn't been that bad before. I spent the rest of the day in bed, but when Dad returned home from work, I think he knew it was more than just an upset stomach.

With my Nan in a much more stable condition, Mum returned from Ireland that evening and first thing the next morning, she took me to see the GP. He didn't hesitate in sending me to A&E, suspecting I had appendicitis. Petrified by the doctor's urgency, we drove straight to A&E where I was immediately admitted to hospital and had my appendix removed that night. Mum said that when I returned from theatre, my skin was almost purple – my appendix must have been on the verge of bursting and she reckons they only just caught it in time.

I've never been so relieved to have medical treatment, although I was still in a lot of pain which was being controlled with morphine. I didn't quite appreciate the strength of that stuff until I awoke in the middle of the night to find myself standing by my bed, still attached to a drip and shouting out for a nurse. I had absolutely no recollection of getting out of bed. God knows I wasn't popular with my fellow patients the next day! I remained in hospital for four days and I hated every minute. The doctors wanted me to stay in for a bit longer, but I begged them to discharge me as soon as I was comfortable enough to walk up the stairs at home. And once again, I was amazed by how much people cared about me as get well cards flooded in each day and people came to visit.

It would take me a while to be fully mobile again and everyone was concerned that if I returned to school and took a fall, I could do more damage to my scar which was still very tender. As it was late November, it was decided that I would stay off school until the New Year. But Year 10 was an important year for my GCSE's and I couldn't afford that much time off school. Mrs Clarke to the rescue!

While I recovered in hospital, she had been attending all my classes, making notes and getting work from the teachers. As soon as I was back at home and feeling stronger, Mrs Clarke started coming to the house each afternoon to in effect, tutor me. She'd got me this far and she wasn't about to let me fall behind. She spent her mornings in my usual lessons and in the afternoon, she'd come over to our house to help me keep up. She truly went above and beyond and it is thanks to her that I returned to school no worse off for my six weeks absence.

That hospital stay wasn't my first and I knew that it wouldn't be my last. Having CP meant I was more familiar than most with hospitals and doctors. Mum and I often joked that we spent half our lives attending appointments. But when I was twelve, it became clear to me why there were so many appointments. My birth had been very traumatic and mistakes had undoubtedly been made. Subsequently, I would always have a physical disability and so Mum and Dad had decided to take legal action against the health board. Many of my hospital appointments helped to build evidence against the hospital and to prove that their negligent actions had caused my disability.

It took over ten years to build the case – yet another ongoing battle for Mum and Dad. I was fourteen when the case finally went to court in March 1998. Mum and Dad were obviously not familiar with court proceedings and nobody advised them on whether or not my attendance would be required. They decided to take me as they thought the case would only take a week. It was a scary but fascinating experience. We met with our lawyers, Damien and Roger, beforehand and they explained the proceedings as best as they could and tried to reassure me. I was only fourteen and I didn't know what to expect. I'd seen court rooms on TV and had almost expected a jury and a dock. But it was the High Court and a civil case so there was just a judge, but still, it was strange seeing all the lawyers in their wigs and I was both nervous and apprehensive as we sat waiting for the case to begin.

I attended court with Mum and Dad for the first few days of the case but the judge had voiced concerns about me being in attendance. He felt that the witness statements and hearing the details of my birth would distress me and on a few occasions he asked me to leave the court and sit outside. Little did the judge realise that as I sat outside the courtroom, I began to get more worried and distressed. After all, I was only fourteen and all these lawyers and barristers were talking and effectively, arguing about me. What were they saying? Did they know things about my future that I was yet to be told? Roger popped out to see me a few times, but I got so anxious, I'd burst into tears. I felt that I was old enough and indeed entitled to hear about what had happened to me and Mum. But it was all getting a bit too much for me and so for the next few days, I stayed with my Nan while Mum and Dad went to court. But nothing could take my mind off what was happening in court and the hours dragged as I waited for Mum and Dad to pick me up and tell me what had been said that day.

Brian visited me after school at my Nan's flat one day, but at this point he didn't know about the court case and Nan let something slip about Mum and Dad being in court. I knew that the case was the first of its kind in Ireland and would probably attract a lot of media interest. I realised it was time to tell him before the media beat me to it. We went for a walk and I began to explain why I was here when I should have been at school. It was the first time I'd talked about any of it with someone my own age and although it was difficult and emotional, it was a relief to let out my feelings and know that I now had my best friend to support me. That night, Mum and Dad took us both out for dinner and it was nice to be distracted from the stress and strain that the court case was causing for us all. From then on, Brian was a great support and helped me cope with the multitude of emotions that I felt over the next few months.

By the end of that week, it became evident that the case was going to drag on and I would miss more crucial time at school. Dad decided he would take me home to Birmingham, while Mum remained in Dublin to follow the case. Once again, Mum was away from the family because of me and I felt so guilty.

As I said, although I'd been aware of the circumstances of my birth, the detail hadn't really bothered me before and I hadn't given it that much thought. But hearing the details and how Mum had feared I was dead absolutely crushed me. I could only imagine Mum and Dad's anguish as they watched the events unfold, but remained powerless to change anything. And that stayed with me for a long time. I wasn't so much angry at the outcome, I was angry at how badly Mum had been treated and at the huge impact on us as a family. I wouldn't change my disability for the world, it's made me who I am and I don't think I've lost out on anything because of it. I have actually always considered myself to be very lucky – my disability could have been much worse. But it couldn't be denied that my life would be harder because of the mistakes the hospital made and now Mum and Dad were being forced to fight to ensure that

I'd always have a good quality of life. I am incredibly grateful to them for fighting so hard for me.

I tried to get on and concentrate on my school work, but my mind was always wandering to what was happening in court. How was Mum coping? What point were the lawyers arguing today? After school, I'd lock myself in my bedroom, put some music on and often have a cry. The case was a huge strain on the family and although I knew that none of this was my fault, I still felt responsible for the stress and strain that we were all feeling.

After three long weeks, Mum and Dad's 25th wedding anniversary was approaching and we all encouraged Dad to go over and spend it with Mum. Although it wasn't the most romantic wedding anniversary, it was certainly their most memorable. That evening they phoned and asked to speak to me. As I took the phone from Collette, I was shaking with nerves and anticipation – were Mum and Dad about to break bad news? Had it all been for nothing? Relief flooded through me as Mum explained that the hospital had decided to settle out of court. The case was over and I had won. The hospital had decided to settle without admitting liability. We didn't care – settling the case was an admission of guilt as far as we were concerned.

As soon as I could, I rang Brian to share the good

news and he promised to tell the gang before the news came on that evening. I was feeling quite overwhelmed by everything and Brian was very supportive, reassuring me that I could now put it all behind me and we could all get on with life. Mum and Dad returned home that weekend and we had a belated party for their anniversary. I was still quite overwhelmed by everything and as well as been incredibly grateful to Mum and Dad, I wanted to thank the legal team for their dedication to the case. I know they were being paid for their efforts, but thanks to their hard work, my future had been made a whole lot easier. So I sat and composed heartfelt thankyou letters to the lawyers, barristers and key witnesses. But no words could really convey the relief and gratitude that I felt and I told them so.

As my 15th birthday approached, I still couldn't shake the feeling of sadness that I'd felt since that first day in court. All I could think about was what I'd heard over the past few weeks – how I'd nearly died and the desperation my parents had felt waiting to hear my first cry. I also wondered about the individuals who were so careless on that day in 1983. Were they even aware of the consequences of their actions? Had they done the same to another mother and child? As I said, I wouldn't change my situation for anything, but that didn't mean that I wanted the same to happen to someone else, to another family. These thoughts bothered me for a long time and I bottled them up, not wanting to burden anyone with my feelings when the case was finally over. But my feelings boiled over one day during a RE lesson. We were talking about the Catholic Church's stance on abortion and someone asked the teacher if abortion would be allowed in a case of cerebral palsy. Although I knew the question was void as CP typically occurs during birth, the case was still fresh in my mind and I sat in that lesson fighting back my tears. It was a difficult few weeks, but I eventually realised that I had to stop dwelling on what had happened in order to move forward.

Word soon got out at school about the case, but nobody asked me any questions and I was soon back to normal. Between my unexpected stay in hospital and the court case, it had been a difficult six months and now I just had two things to concentrate on. Passing my GCSEs and proving my critics wrong.

Chapter 11
Torn

By now, I had a new Headmistress at St. Francis who was Irish and I think that's why I liked her so much. She was always very supportive and I knew she wanted me to achieve as much as I could. I was slightly surprised though when she suggested that I should take just seven GCSEs – Maths, Science, English and English Literature, French, RE and Business Studies. Most of my peers were taking nine or ten, some even more. But the school knew how much effort it took for me just to be at school, let alone study for ten GCSEs. They suggested taking seven would mean that I could really concentrate on those subjects, have some spare study periods and really do my very best. It was a done deal!

Mrs Clarke and I worked harder than we ever had in those final few months and the extra study periods were spent polishing off my coursework and revising for my exams. Although I still needed to put the effort in at home, it took the pressure off me a little bit. It was agreed that as Mrs Clarke had worked with me for so long and understood me so well, she would be allowed to scribe for me during my exams. Although I can only imagine how frustrated she got when she knew I'd got things wrong, but had to write it down anyway! I would search her face for an indication of how she thought I was doing, but she had a brilliant poker face and gave nothing away! Once the exam was over and the paper handed to the teacher who was invigilating, we'd have an autopsy and I'd kick myself as Mrs Clarke told me what she thought I'd got wrong. But I was also reassured to know the things that she thought I'd done well on and that it hadn't been a total disaster!

As I prepared for these final exams of my compulsory education, my thoughts turned once again to my future, which this time, was a little more in my own hands. My hope had been to move into the Sixth Form at St Francis, and with Mrs Clarke's support, complete my A-levels. But it quickly became apparent that the Local Authority would no longer fund Mrs Clarke's position and I would have to continue my education elsewhere. But I couldn't and didn't complain as I'd proven to everyone what I was capable of – I'd lasted five years at St Francis and now here I was, taking my GCSEs.

I now had to decide where to continue my education once my exams were complete. I knew exactly what I wanted to do: A-level English and Business Studies.

English had always been my strongest subject and although I wasn't yet sure about my future career, I figured business skills would always be useful. Even then I knew that one day I wanted to run my own business, so the only decision to make was where I would study. I started looking at local colleges, but they were all unable to provide the support which I knew I would need. Then Mrs Clarke and I met the school's career advisor.

'Have you considered the possibility of applying to a residential college?' I wasn't even aware of their existence, but the advisor went on to explain that there was a college in Coventry specifically for disabled students. As well as offering academic courses, they enabled their students to develop 'life skills' and learn to live independently.

My initial reaction was one of complete reluctance. Mum and Dad had fought so hard to keep me in mainstream education and I had proven that they had been right to fight. How could I now say that I wanted to go a college for disabled people? It went against everything I'd ever known and it felt like I'd be letting Mum and Dad down. But there was a flip side. I'd always been dependent on Mum and Dad for everything and they had been my full-time carers all my life. I had only recently been given an electric wheelchair and I never went further than the local shops without someone with me. I realised as well as studying for my A-levels, I needed to learn to look after myself. This was an opportunity to do that and to finally give Mum and Dad the break that they deserved.

We decided to go and visit the college in Coventry and I think it's fair to say that our first impressions of the college were very good. As well as having a wide range of courses, Hereward College boasted a whole team of Learning Support Workers, an on-site physiotherapist, wheelchair support, as well as adapted accommodation with 24 hour care support. Academic success was obviously important at the college, but equally important was the development of vital life skills – cooking, washing, cleaning and of course, social skills. Not that I needed much help in that department!

As we were shown around the college and introduced to the Principal, my heart was still torn – Mum and Dad had always fought for and looked after me. It felt like I was being ungrateful for wanting to move away and begin a life of my own. But I also knew this was a fantastic opportunity and that if I didn't take it, I would probably never leave home and my parents would always be my carers. As well as wanting more independence, I wanted them to have a life that no longer revolved completely around what was best for me.

So after seeing how well equipped the college was and being very clear about the reasons for my choice, I knew what I had to do. I applied to Hereward College and waited. It would be a fairly lengthy process as even if the college accepted me, I would then need to apply for the funding. So once again, my future was unsettled and I wondered what would happen after I'd completed my exams.

As part of the application process, I was required to attend a two day 'interview' and stay overnight at the college. It was nerve racking, but it gave me a real glimpse into what studying and living at Hereward would be like. During that visit, I still had very mixed feelings. It was exciting being away from home and mixing with people my own age. However, I wasn't used to being around other disabled people, many of whom were much more severely disabled than me and I really didn't know if I'd be able to settle in. As I went to bed that night, my emotions were all over the place. I didn't know what my future held, particularly if I decided that it wasn't for me. None of the local colleges seemed equipped to meet my needs, but Hereward wasn't sitting quite right with me either.

Chapter 12
Fifteen minutes of fame

As a little girl, Mum loved to dress me up in pretty clothes and my wardrobe was full to the brim of frilly, colourful dresses. It wasn't until I was about nine or ten that I even owned a pair of trousers. Mum took great pride in my appearance, but there was always one thing which threatened to overshadow Mum's efforts. My dribbling. Just like a baby, I was constantly drooling and Mum would be forever changing my clothes. If we were going out anywhere, she'd repeat the same instructions, 'Aideen, love, remember to swallow, try not to dribble. It's not nice, love. Here, take this tissue.'

Embarrassment and shame would engulf me even though I knew that Mum's plea wasn't about saving her own embarrassment, but about saving mine. She wasn't scolding me or trying to make me feel bad. She just knew that people already saw me as 'different' and didn't want them having more reason to stare and point. I'd automatically reply with something like, 'Yes Mum, I'll try.' But I knew it wasn't that simple. For one, I wasn't always aware that I was dribbling until my chest got so damp that it looked like I'd been caught in the rain without a mac. It's always been difficult for me to concentrate on more than one thing at a time and if I was trying my damnedest to walk in a straight line, also remembering to swallow regularly was near on impossible. My brain just couldn't send two signals at once. And secondly, I didn't want to spend all my time worrying about something that was so difficult for me to control. If Mum was with me, she'd do her best to remind me to swallow as discreetly as she could. But Mum couldn't be with me all the time. In my mind, I was just a normal little girl and as such, I didn't have a single care in the world. I was just Aideen and naivety told me that people should just accept me as I was.

But as I grew up and into a teenager, that naivety melted away and I realised that a cruel, judgemental world awaited me. As hormones kicked in and boys consumed my thoughts, I began to realise that appearances mattered. A lot. All the boys went for the girls with short skirts, shaved legs and pretty faces. The sad reality dawned that very few lads, if any, would even glance in my direction with my spotty face, wet chin and hairy legs. I became very self-conscience about my dribbling, but as much as I tried to control it, I was fighting a losing battle.

One evening, Mum was watching a documentary about someone who had had a procedure that reversed the salivary glands so that more saliva would be swallowed rather than dribbled. Mum wondered whether the same could be done for me and at my next hospital check-up, she mentioned it to my consultant. Although they didn't do it at my local hospital, I could be referred to Birmingham Children's Hospital to talk it through with the specialist consultant, Mr Proops. After meeting him, he agreed that I'd be an ideal candidate for the operation and that it could really benefit me. The operation was scheduled for just after my GCSEs in June.

I didn't like hospitals or operations, but I liked Mr Proops and he put me at ease. The end of my exams would be bitter sweet, but then something totally unexpected happened. I was contacted by the BBC. They had heard about my approaching operation and they wondered if I would be prepared to appear on Children's Hospital? I didn't take much persuading – I was dreading the operation, but starring on TV would make it all that much more bearable! As if I wasn't convinced, the BBC wanted to film the introduction at Drayton Manor, a local theme park, and I would be allowed to bring along a few friends to celebrate the end of our exams! Perfect distraction from the thoughts of what was ahead.

We enjoyed a brilliant day at Drayton Manor – I've always been a dare devil. As Mum says, the bigger the ride, the happier I am! The BBC crew filmed and interviewed us and when they had enough footage, they joined us on the rides. It gave the viewers an insight into who I was and why I was having the operation. I remember one of the crew members was quite good looking and I developed a bit of a crush on him. Having him around made it all worthwhile! Although I was also a little embarrassed that he'd be filming my operation and seeing me all groggy and out of it afterwards.

The morning of the operation dawned and Mum and I made our way into Birmingham Children's Hospital. Dad was working and would come and see me after the operation that evening. As always, I was terrified. Having general anaesthetic always scared me and once I was settled on the ward, I made Mr Proops explain again and again how safe I would be, how long I would be out for (not that it really made a difference to me) and that he would look after me. Mum promised to be there when I woke up and so as the cameras continued to roll, I was wheeled down to theatre. The anaesthetic went into one hand as Mum held the other and counted ten, nine, eight... And I was gone!

I woke up relieved that it was over and Mr Proops (and the crew) told me how well things had gone. I'd have to stay in hospital for one night and providing I felt well enough, I would be discharged the next day. The crew were now gone and I wouldn't see them again until my check-up appointment in six weeks' time.

Mum collected me the next day, but my recovery was only just beginning. During the operation, Mr Proops had clamped my tongue and mouth to keep it open. As a result, I had a mouth full of ulcers and I was in agony. I hadn't been warned about this bit and I was glad the cameras weren't around as I felt so miserable. It was a week before I could eat anything – my new found freedom from school wasn't getting off to a great start. Hungry and in agony! I remember Brian phoning to see how I was, but I could barely speak to him, it hurt so much.

I didn't regret having the operation – it was after all my choice and I knew the pain would be worth it in the end. I was sixteen and starting to turn my attention to lads and possibly finding my first real boyfriend. The results of the operation would hopefully give me more confidence, though I'm sure you're convinced that I was confident enough!

The programme wasn't broadcast until a few months after the operation and it was certainly very strange watching the procedure, knowing it was my big mouth that I was looking at! I realised why I had been in so much pain, as my mouth had been held wide open with several clamps and fingers. As was always the case, I hated listening to my own voice as it sounds so slow and disjointed, but apart from that, I enjoyed my fifteen minutes of fame. Not least because I hoped that by seeing my experience, it might help other people to realise what medical interventions were possible to help them have a better quality of life.

As I slowly recovered from my operation, my thoughts turned towards my GCSE results. They were due out at the end of August – the same day as my follow up appointment with Mr Proops. I was nervous and excited as Mum drove me to the school. The Bridge Hall, as it was called, was heaving with pupils, parents and teachers, but I eventually tracked down my envelope and tore it open. There were pupils all around me, most crying with relief or disappointment and Mum was looking at me expectantly. My eyes misted and I cracked a huge smile as I showed her the piece of paper which displayed three A's, two B's and four C's. Mum squealed with delight and we both cried. The fight had been well worth the effort and I'd achieved what I set out to do five years earlier, I'd silenced my critics – and my God, it felt amazing! English had always been my strongest subject and I'd got A for English Literature and a double B for English Language. I'd also secured Grade A in Business Studies. I now had what I needed to enrol on my chosen A-levels.

Still on a high, our next stop was home to deliver the good news to Dad. He was as proud and as happy as

Mum had been. They had both always told me that I could only do my best and as long as I gave my best, they were happy. I don't think even they expected me to bag three A's and it made victory all the sweeter to exceed even their high expectations of me. As we headed to the hospital for my follow up appointment, Mum couldn't wait to tell anyone who would listen about how well I'd done. Just as well that the BBC crew were filming my follow up appointment – she could tell the whole nation and she did! As I'd done so well and Mum wasn't afraid to shout about it, I think it helped to get the message across that disabled people aren't dumb, they do have brains and with the right support, we can achieve much more than a lot of people might expect.

It had taken a lot of soul searching to decide finally that Hereward College was the right choice for my further education. But as well as completing my A-levels, I would be able to develop the skills that I would need to be able to live independently in the future. Although I still felt very apprehensive about the prospect of moving away from mainstream education, I also knew that the college was the only place which could provide me with the right support to continue my studies.

Now that I had my results, I knew that Hereward was within my sights. It seemed to take forever for the funding to be confirmed, but as soon as it was in place,

Mum and I set about preparing for my first term in Coventry. I was once again anxious and nervous – my next big challenge lay ahead of me and it involved leaving home for the first time. Yes, it was only 30 minutes away and I would come home at weekends, but I was still spreading my wings and learning to fly. I was excited, anxious, happy and sad all at the same time. No doubt Mum and Dad were feeling all of those emotions too and more.

The car was packed and we all piled in. Only we weren't going on a family holiday. It was early in September 1999 and I was heading for Coventry – my first home from home. The whole family wanted to come and see me settled in my new pad but I also think they all wanted to make sure I'd stay in Coventry! As I said, the college was only half an hour from our home in Great Barr, but this was a big step for me and therefore it was a big deal for everyone.

When we arrived on that Sunday afternoon, the college was bustling with excited students and their no doubt anxious families. There were three residential blocks and I was allocated my room on C Block – a small single room which was a bit tired-looking, but clean and cosy and I soon made it feel like home with my posters, books and my treasured teddy bear which Brian brought me back from one of his family holidays.

While everyone helped me to unpack, it gave my family an opportunity to get used to this new chapter in my life. While I was excited about my new adventure, I was acutely aware of Mum's reluctance to leave me. She'd always cared for me, we'd always been together and I knew how hard it was for her to let me go. Although I know that Dad felt the same, he's always been a little more pragmatic. He could see that I was ready for my independence and that Hereward could give me that, while also offering the support that I needed.

One of the care staff noticed how difficult Mum was finding it and she made a promise to her to look out for me. Her name was Mo, she was a mum herself, and could fully relate to how my Mum was feeling. It was Mo's reassurances that eventually gave her the confidence to leave me.

As I watched my family pile back into the car, I suddenly felt very lonely and the tears welled in my eyes. Mum and Dad reassured me that if I was unhappy or couldn't settle, they would come and collect me. I nearly asked them to take me home there and then, but I knew I had to give it a chance if I was ever going to live independently. That didn't stop my heart breaking as my family drove away without me.

Chapter 13
Flying the nest

As soon as my family had pulled away, I headed back to my room to try and compose myself. It was time for me to grow up and spread my wings, but I was still only sixteen. This was going to take time. Because of my mainstream education, I hadn't really spent much time with other disabled people and I wasn't really sure how I would settle in. The college catered for a wide range of students and their disabilities varied a lot in severity – some were a lot more able than me and others were much more severe and really did require 24 hour care and support. This worried me a little – I didn't want or need the care staff to do more than I needed them to and I wondered how I would establish my independence now I was away from home.

The care team had three shifts – morning, afternoon and night. At the beginning of the morning and afternoon shifts, the staff were allocated their students who they would support to get up in the morning or to go to bed at night. As soon as we knew which care worker we had been allocated, there would be a scramble to get in first and book the latest possible bed time. Within days, the care team realised how independent I was and I no longer 'booked' a time. The staff just looked in on me before their shift ended and on nights when I was feeling particularly tired, they took my wheelchair to the charging bay for me.

My first night away from home was inevitably quite strange. I wasn't on a sleep over or away for a week in Lourdes. This was my first home from home and within days I began to wonder if I'd made the right decision. Although the staff encouraged independence, I was told that I wasn't allowed to lock my door at night and with so many people around, people I didn't yet know, it felt like my privacy wasn't a top priority.

Then I met my personal tutor, Dick. He was a lovely man and I took to him immediately. He introduced us newbies to the current students and mentioned something about 'the next three years.' I panicked. Three years? A-level courses were only meant to take two years and that's what I'd been planning for. As soon as Dick dismissed the class, I stayed behind to talk to him. I explained that I had been under the impression that the course would take two years. During the whole application process, nobody had ever mentioned three years. Dick was a little surprised but also sympathetic as he explained that three years was the norm at Hereward as they offered a slower pace of learning in order to cater for all students. I was convinced that I could complete the course in two years, but Dick was equally convinced that Hereward's structure would make it a three year course.

I was gutted. Mum and Dad had sent me to mainstream school to ensure that I'd always be pushed and fulfil my true potential. My main reason for choosing Hereward had been the opportunity to develop my independence – not for a slower working pace. I had already proved that I was bright and could manage in a mainstream environment and now it was becoming clear that Hereward wasn't going to challenge me academically as I had hoped. It felt like I was taking a huge step backwards and as I tried to settle in, that troubled me.

As the lectures for Business Studies began, I realised that we would be given bite size information during lectures and then complete the relevant assignment. The next lecture would be provided when everybody was at the same point. Although there were only six of us, we all worked at very different paces and I felt like I was being spoon fed. We weren't set any work to complete between lectures and the structure of the course made it difficult for me to get on with work independently. I felt frustrated, but my decision had been made and I knew I'd just have to get on with things.

In those first few weeks away from home, I was keen to grab my independence. I'd never really been out on my own as Mum would fret about me and my school friends were often busy doing their own thing. So my first trip out felt like real freedom! I signed myself out of the block and off I went to the local shops. A fairly boring trip, but it felt good finally being able to go out and have time to myself.

Only things didn't quite go to plan. I was on my way back and was about five hundred yards from the college when my wheelchair suddenly stopped. Cut dead. My first solo trip and my chair lets me down! Now what was I supposed to do? It was another occasion when I was thankful that I had a level of mobility. I got out of my chair and checked all the connections. Nothing I did worked. The chair was dead. I switched my attention to Plan B. I put the wheelchair in manual and began pushing it back. I must have looked a right sight trying to push it, keep my balance and steer the chair! I made it back to base and got help. I'd certainly never forget my first solo trip.

Chapter 14
Burnt pasta bake

I soon got to know my class mates and the other students on my block and I soon realised that there was a whole new side to Hereward which I hadn't really considered before: dating!

I'd never had a proper boyfriend before. I'd had many childish crushes on lads, but I'd never received any attention – and no, Austin doesn't count! So I was excited and a bit embarrassed to receive a bouquet of flowers from one of the lads on the other block. I was very flattered, but unfortunately I didn't return this lad's affections. But still he persisted and eventually I agreed to 'go out' with him.

It was probably the first time I'd given into peer pressure. Everyone else in the college seemed to be dating and I didn't want to be boring. But I was also craving 'normality' – to be like any other teenage girl and enjoy the attention that I was finally getting. But I didn't enjoy it and although I liked this lad's company, he didn't make my stomach flutter and if I'm honest, I think I felt sorry for him. He seemed to have a lot of problems and looking back, I wanted to help him. But I soon realised that I wasn't happy and after just a few weeks, I ended the 'relationship'. I was young and knew very little about real relationships, but I knew they shouldn't make you as unhappy as I seemed to be with him.

Part of the problem was that I'd taken a particular shine to one chap on my GNVQ Course. You probably won't believe me, but his name was also Dean! He had been at the college for a few years and was working hard to try and complete his course. I'd secretly liked him for weeks but, as was my past experience, the lads I liked never seemed to return my feelings and so I kept quiet. I think eventually our mutual friends worked out how I felt and knew how unhappy I'd been during my first dating experience. The college was a very close knit community and my little crush eventually became known to Dean.

Eventually, Dean asked me out and he became my first proper boyfriend! (A boyfriend for a few weeks doesn't really count, right?) I was thrilled – I was finally growing up and my confidence was soaring at last. Our first date was to McDonald's, but I didn't care! For the first time ever, the lad I liked had returned my affections and it felt brilliant to be like any normal sixteen-year old. Although I now enjoyed a good social life, I was still very focused on my studies and that always came first.

Though I was confident enough in myself, I'd always found it difficult to imagine finding a boyfriend who would accept me for who I was, four wheels and all. Dean also had CP and I think it was a refreshing confidence boost for me to find a guy I liked who didn't care about my disability. Dean and I seemed to complement each other – we both used electric wheelchairs, but whereas I could walk, albeit not very far, Dean couldn't walk at all. But unlike me, Dean's speech wasn't affected by his CP. We balanced each other well.

During the summer term came my first ever Prom and I was extremely excited that I had a date to share it with! I went shopping for a new dress and when the day finally arrived, I spent hours getting ready with the help of the care staff. My hair was curled and my make-up neatly applied. I felt like a princess as I waited for Dean to pick me up, as he had insisted on doing. He arrived with a single red rose and a cuddly bear to sweep me off my feet! It was the perfect start to a wonderful evening and that night is one of my happiest memories of my Hereward days. My disability was irrelevant; I was just a young, love-struck teenager enjoying one of her first ever dates.

After a very shaky start, both academically and personally, that first year of college was brilliant. I finally had my independence and my relationship with

Dean made me so happy. But not everyone was quite so happy. Not only was Mum adjusting to me not being at home, she had to get used to the fact that I was now a young lady with a boyfriend. And she made her disapproval very clear! Although Dean was just five years older than me, Mum thought he was too old for me and would only distract me from my studies. At the time, it frustrated me that Mum disapproved so much and we did clash whenever Dean came up! But looking back on it now, I know that Mum was just worried about me as she came to realise that she could no longer protect me from everything.

My first year at Hereward drew to a close and as well as being so happy, I'd also done well academically. Although Dean would be leaving half way into my second year, I was looking forward to returning in September.

Only I got a bit of a surprise when I arrived at the beginning of term. Instead of having a standard single room, I had been given what they called the 'Training Flat'. It was on the residential block, but I'd have my own space including my own kitchen, bedroom and bathroom! The care staff had realised how independent I was and this was an opportunity for me to further develop my independence in preparation for the future.

I didn't wait too long to make the most of my

independence and one evening, I decided to make a pasta bake for my dinner. Simple enough, right? Wrong. I managed to burn the pasta and set the fire alarm off, which automatically called the fire brigade! I had the whole college in a panic and I was so embarrassed. I couldn't even do pasta bake and I was the butt of many jokes for days. Let's just say I opted to eat in the canteen from then on!

The care staff were still available 24 hours a day should I need them, but nonetheless, the flat gave me a taste of independent living and really gave me confidence in my own abilities. With a little help, I began to feel confident that I could manage to look after myself at university even though that was still a year away.

During that second year at Hereward, Dean finished his course and returned home. I was heartbroken and my life became a constant countdown to the next time we'd see each other. We'd agreed to have a long distance relationship, but looking back now it was a bad idea. We'd already had some silly rows and split up once while in college. Though I wouldn't admit it then, our relationship wasn't strong enough to overcome the difficulties of distance and separation. I don't think either of us realised we were both too young for a long-term commitment.

But nonetheless, we remained together, spending

hours on the phone each evening and Dean would return to Hereward to visit me whenever he could. It wasn't the same, but we were utterly determined, as young people often are, to stay together.

In the meantime, as my second year at Hereward was coming to a close, Mum and Dad had made a big decision. They were selling our house in Great Barr and moving back to Sligo (though they later also bought a smaller house in Great Barr, so they could come and go as they pleased). They had been toying with the idea for a few years and had finally found a house in Sligo that they liked. They had secured a school place for James and in July 2001, we all said a sad goodbye to what had been my childhood home. It held so many memories for us all and as we packed up and drove away, it's one of the few times I've seen my Dad tearful.

Mum and Dad's decision to move back to Ireland left me with a big decision of my own. I knew that they wanted me to go with them and they had found a specialist disabled college in Sandymount, near Dublin. We'd gone to visit the college, but it wasn't a patch on Hereward and it didn't have any residential accommodation. I had already completed my English A-level and had done so much work for the GNVQ. I knew that I couldn't throw all that away and although Dean was now at home, I didn't really want to put any further distance between us. As difficult as it was for all of us, I decided I would return to Hereward in September and finish what I'd started.

But what then? I knew my Mum wanted me to join the family in Ireland and my heart was torn. The whole family were now there, except for me. But in terms of accessibility, Ireland was trailing behind the UK. Our home town of Sligo wasn't very accessible and there were no wheelchair friendly buses or taxis. I'd be even more reliant on Mum and Dad than I had been in Birmingham and I knew that long-term, I'd have a better chance of building a career in the UK.

So without telling anyone, I started applying for universities in the UK and I picked out six which offered the course I wanted as well as offering good support for disabled students. It wasn't that I wanted to keep it from my family, but I just wasn't ready and didn't know how to tell them that I wasn't moving to Ireland.

I went to visit several universities, but it was Mrs Clarke who, once again, guided me towards Oxford Brookes University. She had heard that it had an excellent Disabled Student Advice department and after researching as much as I could, I decided to put in an application and select it as my first choice. It had a brilliant reputation and even though my heart was already set on it, I doubted whether they would accept me. It gave me the motivation to work that bit harder during my final months at Hereward.

I anxiously awaited a letter from UCAS, the Universities and Colleges Admissions Service, to tell me which universities, if any, had offered me a place. I was overjoyed when it finally arrived – five out of the six universities had offered me a conditional place! Including Oxford Brookes! I thought back, as I often do, to those kids in the playground who had said I wouldn't manage a week in our new school. If they could only see this piece of paper.

Now came the hard part. Telling my family that I was going to university in the UK. I braced myself for a lot of upset and I decided to tell Dad first. I was at home in Sligo for the holidays and my mouth was dry as I explained to him that I'd applied to UCAS and had been conditionally accepted into Oxford Brookes. I was worried he'd be disappointed that I hadn't consulted anybody and might even be angry. But there was none of that. Dad completely understood and supported my decision to stay in the UK, he knew my life there was settled and that I'd have more opportunities over there. I explained that Oxford Brookes had an excellent reputation for supporting disabled students and he could see I'd done my research. I was so pleased Dad accepted and supported my decision, but I was worried about Mum. She only ever wanted the best for me and when I was away from her, nothing would stop her worrying. But

Ireland couldn't offer me what I needed, so Dad offered to talk to Mum about Oxford Brookes.

I'm not sure what he said to her, but the next time they came to see me at Hereward, they suggested we drive down to Oxford to have a look around. I can only imagine how difficult it was for Mum as I could see the anxiety on her face. She was slowly letting me go, letting me grow up, but I knew we would always be close. After our trip to Oxford, we all knew it was ideal and although Dean would have also liked me to be closer to him, he too accepted that Brookes was the best option for me. With the support of my nearest and dearest, my heart was truly set on Brookes and I worked hard to ensure that I got there.

Chapter 15
Two sheets to the wind

When I look back at my time at Hereward, I have a mixed view. On one hand, it left me very frustrated academically. I was constantly being spoon fed, most of my exams were multi choice questions and I don't remember ever feeling under pressure or challenged academically in any way. I know now that I thrive under pressure and I absolutely love a challenge – the bigger the challenge, the more motivated I am.

On the other hand, I know that I wouldn't be where I am today without my experience at Hereward. Moving away from home at the tender age of sixteen was ultimately my decision and one which I'm sure my Mum thought I wasn't ready to make. But I often wonder, when would Mum have been ready for me to leave home? The answer is that I'd probably still be there. Mum sometimes joked that she would build me a 'granny flat' in her garden and that scared me because I knew there was an element of seriousness in her suggestion. I wanted and needed my freedom, but more importantly, I didn't want to be a burden to Mum and Dad for the rest of their lives. I wanted us to have a normal parent/child relationship as I grew into an adult.

Hereward was both a compromise and a stepping stone. It gave me the skills and confidence I needed to build an independent life, but also, I hope, gave Mum the security of knowing that there was support available if I needed it. Without Hereward, there would have been no chance of me taking my next big step - living independently in Halls of Residence.

I was about to start a new adventure in Oxford and although I was excited, I was equally terrified. There would be no carers on call 24/7 and for the first time ever, I'd be responsible for absolutely everything – paying rent and bills, cooking, washing, getting to and from lectures as well as studying for my degree. It was a huge change for me and as Mum and Dad drove away, I remember feeling very lonely. Only it felt different to when they'd left me at Hereward and I was full of self-doubt. The full-time support network at Hereward had given me the skills and the confidence to get to where I was now. Oxford Brookes had an excellent reputation for supporting disabled students, but I still felt vulnerable without the back-up of 24-hour support.

Nonetheless, I couldn't fault the support that was put in place by the Disability Support Team. Firstly, they arranged for me to have a note taker in all of my lectures and somebody to scribe for me during exams. Most of the people who supported me were brilliant and I was so grateful for their help. On occasions, I got matched with people who weren't so good and that was difficult. As I wasn't employing my support workers myself, it wasn't my place to reprimand them if they were late or not taking full notes. It could be frustrating and on one occasion, I had to request a different support worker because I was repeatedly being let down.

Although strictly speaking it wasn't their responsibility, the Team also arranged for someone to come and help me in my Halls of Residence, twice a week. This was mainly so that Mum could rest easy, knowing that I was getting a decent meal at least twice a week! It also gave me a bit of a break and usually, the support worker would cook enough food for a couple of days.

As well as the normal Student Loan, I received a grant from the LEA to cover the cost of any equipment which would help me to complete my degree. The Disability Team organised a laptop for me and even found a specialist company to make a custom key guard for it. I cannot tell you how useful it was as it saved me spending hours doing coursework in the IT suites, which didn't have any specialist computer equipment.

With all this fantastic support now in place, I threw myself into university life and soon found my feet. I was given a place in Halls of Residence, not far from the main university campus. I'd be sharing with four other students in one of the wheelchair accessible flats. Only moving in with four complete strangers wasn't plain sailing and took a lot of getting used to. One of the other students was also a wheelchair user and even though she was much more capable than me, she had a live-in carer. Up until this point, she'd been an only child living at home with her parents and she had a set routine which she wasn't prepared, or perhaps able, to change. Her ideas about student life were very different to ours and within weeks, it was causing arguments. She'd go to bed at 9 pm on the dot and then expect us to turn down our TVs and music. If we did what students do and went out drinking, we'd be told off for waking her up when we came home a bit worse for wear. It became quite tiresome that she always wanted things her way, particularly as she had no problem getting up at 6 am and waking us.

But not liking tension, I often found myself in the role of peace keeper between her and the two lads who shared with us. I got on very well with Ron and Harris and despite the tension in the flat, we made the most of being freshers! As lectures began, I settled into a routine of my own, but no matter how hard I tried, I couldn't shift the loneliness that I'd felt as Mum and

Dad had left. Although Ron and Harris became good friends, I felt like an outsider on my course and whenever we were required to work in groups, there was never a natural choice for me. Each time I worked in a group, I'd hope to meet people who might become friends, but they never did. As soon as our assignment had been completed, the only time I'd see them was in lectures.

This was the same throughout my first and second year. Don't get me wrong, I had lots of nights out with Ron and Harris and my second year flatmates and at times, I lived up to the typical student lifestyle! But I just couldn't seem to click with anyone else on my course, so if I was struggling with an assignment or just needed someone to bounce ideas off, I had nobody to talk to. Whereas the other students would wait around for their friends after a lecture, I'd hurry off to get the bus home.

I went through a really difficult few months and I felt so lonely. Dean wasn't able to come and see me very often and although he phoned every day, it wasn't the same. He was miles away and my family were in another country. I felt like a little girl lost in a big city. At times, when I felt at my worst, I wondered whether I'd even see my Graduation Day. I was at my lowest when I decided to go and see my personal tutor. I didn't really expect her to do anything, but I was desperate just to talk to someone about how I was feeling. I was blown away by her response. She inquired if I had any hobbies and told me about a disabled sailing club that she knew about. She insisted on taking me one evening and I had a wonderful time. It gave me a break from my studies and the boost that I needed. Unfortunately, the club was about thirty minutes away from my flat and I couldn't get there on my own, but I've never forgotten that lady's kindness. Another who went way beyond the call of duty!

Although it wasn't practical for me to take up sailing, I knew it was time to take matters into my own hands and find an interest that would provide me with a break from my studies. I began wandering around the Student Union and even thought that I might find a part-time job. With this in mind, I went into the JobShop. The lady who ran it was called Sue and I instantly liked her. Although Sue didn't really have any jobs which would be suitable for me, we chatted away like old friends and she was sympathetic to my situation. From then on, I regularly popped in for a natter. I'd suddenly found a friend in the unlikeliest of places and I was so grateful. In time, I started to help out there and it gave me a break from my studies.

Spending so much time in the Student Union also opened up other opportunities. The Student Union needed a Disability Officer and with Sue's encouragement, I decided to stand for the position and a few weeks later, I was elected. Before discovering the JobShop, I'd felt so lonely and isolated that I wanted to make a difference for other disabled students who might be feeling the same and it would be a way for me to make new friends.

From that point on, my loneliness disappeared as I threw myself into Student Union life and got to know a whole bunch of new people. I did my best to represent and engage with all disabled students and even attended a national conference in Blackpool, but it was a difficult role. Perhaps disabled students didn't like the thought of being grouped together and although I continued to try and engage them, I'm not sure I had much of an impact if I'm honest. But I made myself available and students knew I was there to help and represent them if need be.

Now before I continue, you need to understand something:

As soon as I was old enough to drink, (my 18th birthday, of course!) I had an amazing revelation that was to change my life for the better. Alcohol was good for me. Seriously. The more alcohol I drank, the less severe by spasms became and the clearer my speech was. I'd start the night completely unable to hold my drink without spilling it and by my third drink, I could bring the glass to my mouth without so much as a thought! It was amazing - alcohol chilled me out completely. I know that's what it's meant to do, but for me the effects were quite beneficial.

Now don't get me wrong. I know I'm Irish, but I'm not an alcoholic. I just enjoy a drink. Or two. OK, OK, maybe quite a few! And my Student Union days gave me the perfect opportunity to do just that. After all, I was expected to be a role model for other disabled students and I had to show them how to have a good time! One of the perks of being a student officer was getting on the Guest List for all the big party nights. I'd drag my flatmates along, not that they needed much dragging... We'd drink and dance the nights away until we got kicked out of the union. That's when I was always grateful that there was no law against being drunk in charge of a wheelchair, although perhaps there should have been! On one occasion, I was walking home with one of my fellow Student Union officers and I was walking (you know what I mean!) on the footpath, nearest to the road. As we drunkenly chatted away, I lost all concentration and all of a sudden, I was lying sideways in my chair - in the middle of the road. I'd fallen off the footpath! Luckily, it was two-thirty in the morning, the road was dead and I completely escaped injury. My friend helped me to get the wheelchair upright again and although we laughed about it, I knew I'd been lucky.

On another occasion, as I made my way back to my Halls of Residence, again a little worse for wear, I passed a police car that was stationary at some traffic lights. Being a friendly person, I started waving profusely at the police officers as I crossed the road in front of them. I'm sure it was obvious that I was two sheets to the wind, but seeing that I was safely across the road, the officers simply waved back and continued their patrol.

University life was finally going well and I was getting into a good routine. Though a carer popped in twice a week to help out, I slowly became relatively independent. Whenever possible, I'd get a meal in the university canteen and then eat a lighter meal in the evening. The Team had arranged for my flat to have a washing machine and a tumble dryer put in so that I didn't have to traipse with all my washing to the on-site launderette.

The only problem was travelling to and from the campus in Wheatley where most of my lectures were delivered. The university laid on its own bus which operated quite regularly and as the bus was accessible, it enabled me to make the twenty minute journey. Except at peak times, when the bus was jam packed, I had absolutely no hope of getting on it with my wheelchair. It was one thing getting on the bus, but it was quite another trying to position the wheelchair in its required designated space. I loved the independence of catching the bus when it was quiet, but when it was busy it became extremely irritating as I repeatedly had to wait for the next bus in the hope that there would be space for me on that one.

Eventually, after many frustrating mornings stranded at the bus stop, I mentioned it to the Disability Support Team and they arranged a tab for me with a local taxi firm so that I could get a taxi at times when I knew the bus would be too busy. It was a major relief and I soon had a regular driver who I could phone whenever I needed to get over to Wheatley, though I was careful not to abuse it. If I was going further than usual, I made up the difference myself and I never offered lifts to other students, unless they were supporting me in lectures.

Although university life was busy, I always found time for flying my kite and having fun! It was my cousin's twenty-first birthday and I was going over to Dublin for her party. It would be a flying visit as I was busy studying, so I was arriving on the Friday, the night of the party, and leaving again on the Sunday. I was staying with my best friend Brian and we were both going to the party.

But when I landed at Dublin airport, disaster struck. The airline had lost my luggage and with only a few hours until the party, I didn't think I'd have anything to wear! I left Brian's address with the staff and, given the circumstances, they promised to track down my bag and courier it out to me as soon as possible. In the meantime, my friends rallied to see what they could lend me, just in case. With an hour to go, my luggage arrived and we were all looking forward to the party once again.

Our Family parties always go with a bang and this one wasn't going to be any different! As the main party came to a close, a few of us decided to continue in the hotel's nightclub. My cousin Gerard, Brian and myself headed down to the club entrance, fully expecting to join other friends and family who had gone ahead of us. For some reason, I'd walked down to the club with Brian's support rather than be in my manual wheelchair. We waited in the queue like everyone else, but when we got to the top it, the bouncer said we weren't allowed in and ushered other people passed us. We'd had a few drinks, but we weren't being rowdy – we'd just been chatting in the queue. When we asked why we couldn't go in, the bouncer said the strobe lighting in the club would affect me. I couldn't believe my ears! He hadn't even spoken to me and yet he'd made a judgement about my condition. But I have cerebral palsy, not epilepsy and I told him so, but he wouldn't listen to me or the lads.

After a few minutes of trying to put our point across, the bouncer then said I wasn't allowed in as there wasn't a female with me to assist me to go to the toilet! Another wild assumption he'd made without even talking to me. I was perfectly capable of going to the toilet alone, but again, he didn't care and I was furious. Without even uttering a word to me, he assumed he knew everything about my condition, when in fact he knew nothing. The lads had been calm and reasonable to start with, but now they were furious and at one point, I thought Brian was going to punch him, so I pulled him away.

When one of my female cousins arrived, the bouncer suddenly did a U-turn and agreed to let us in, but by that time, I didn't want to give them a penny of my money and we went home fuming. Although Brian is my best friend, we don't see each other that much and so Brian hadn't ever really experienced anything like that before and I think he was as angry as I was.

The experience ruined my weekend – it was the 21st century and yet such stupid, bloody ignorance still existed. My anger didn't subside and I made a complaint through my solicitor. Unfortunately, the law is an ass and I didn't get very far, although all I'd wanted was an apology and an acknowledgement that they were in the wrong.

Chapter 16

Suited and booted

I was suited and booted and ready to impress. It was the second year of my Business Management degree at Oxford Brookes University and my third year would be spent on a paid work placement. I'd chosen a four year sandwich course for a reason. I knew finding employment would be a challenge – I'd have to convince potential employers that my disability didn't equal inability and that I was very capable of holding down a job. I thought a year of experience on my CV would help me secure a role upon graduation. Little did I realise that I was about to get my first real dose of discrimination.

After several failed applications, I'd managed to bag an interview with a small marketing company near Oxford and the job sounded perfect for me. The interview went really well – I'd been grilled by just two people, but I felt I'd come across really well and they'd responded quite positively to me. I came out feeling fairly confident – this could be the one, I thought to myself. A few days later my confidence was in tatters as I read an email from the Managing Director (MD) of the company. He stated quite bluntly that he couldn't possibly employ me as his clients wouldn't be able to communicate with me. Why? Because his clients wouldn't be able to understand my speech.

He hadn't faulted my skills or my abilities compared to other candidates. That was his one and only reason for rejecting me. I was fuming! Who was he to judge whether his clients would be able to understand me? I know my speech isn't *that* difficult to understand as I successfully communicate with people on a daily basis. I knew I couldn't just let this go so after a few hours of seething, I decided to sit down and compose a polite reply to the MD. I told him it was a shame he felt the way he did as he'd dismissed a huge asset to his team. I continued that there were many ways of communicating with clients and that if every employer were to have his views, I would sadly remain unemployed. My aim wasn't to get him to change his mind, but to educate him. I made sure to come across as super confident, even a little arrogant, though inside my confidence had been snatched away from me.

A few days later, I received another email which listed seven or eight reasons why I had not been appointed. It was obvious the MD had cobbled the list together and if the reasons had been genuine, why hadn't he just given me that list in the first place? If he genuinely thought another candidate was better than me and had evidence to prove it, then why even bring my disability into it? His delayed explanation was just a cover in case I decided to take a case against him. But what would be the point? I wouldn't want to work for him now anyway and I think I'd got my point across quite effectively!

The experience made me realise the extent of discrimination that disabled people face and I knew I wanted to do something about it. But I still struggled to find a placement. I spent hours filling in application forms and tweaking my CV so that it was relevant for each position that I applied for. But I still struggled to secure any interviews. One of the few interviews which I did get, for a logistics role, was pretty much ruined by an ignorant taxi driver. Even though I booked the taxi in advance and with plenty of time before my interview, the driver turned up really late. Not seeming to care much for my inconvenience, he bundled me into his black cab. But worse was to come when we arrived at the company. Firstly, the driver decided to drop me off in the middle of the road, rather than taking the time to find a safe, suitable place to drop me off. Then, as I wheeled my chair out of his cab, my wheels messed up a mat that he had on the floor of his cab and he decided to have a go at me! I was absolutely furious with his attitude, but as I was about to go for an interview, I had to try and keep calm. Any other time and I'd have given him a piece of my mind, but I was worried about the impression that might have given the interviewers, on top of me being late. Needless to say though, I was wound up and although the interview went ok, I didn't get the position.

Christmas was fast approaching and despite making dozens of applications, I still hadn't secured a placement. I was starting to worry, as most of my peers had been successful and were free to focus on the end of year exams and assignments. However, I had a trip of a lifetime coming up which would temporarily distract me from my growing concerns. I was going to Australia with Mum, Dad and James to visit my sister Martina, who was now based in Melbourne. I was hugely excited to be getting away from it all and hoped that the trip would give me a fresh perspective on things.

I was going for almost six weeks so my flat mates suggested some farewell drinks the night before my trip. Any excuse for students to drink! But things took a sinister turn when, after just one drink, I began feeling light headed and a bit out of control. I put it down to end-of-term stress and tiredness. But after a few sips of my second drink, I knew it was more than tiredness, the room was spinning and I could barely lift my head. My flatmate, Nahid, helped me back to my room and into bed and then confessed that the lads had been adding extra vodka to my drinks, a lot extra it seemed. Normally, I might have been amused, but I was going to Australia tomorrow and now I'd be nursing a massive hangover. I was absolutely furious with the boys but reprimands would have to wait until the morning. Luckily we had an evening flight, but I had to make my own way to Heathrow; I wasn't looking forward to that now.

The next day, the boys got the sharp end of my tongue, but after grovelling apologies, I finished my packing and made my way to the bus stop. Hangover or not, I couldn't be late meeting Mum and Dad and somehow, I would have to try and hide the fact that I was suffering! Despite such an awful start, we had an absolutely amazing holiday. After spending Christmas in Melbourne, we spent the next few weeks travelling up the East Coast of Australia, taking in Sydney, Brisbane, the Gold Coast and finally, Cairns. I ticked off another first by going snorkelling at the Great Barrier Reef, which was absolutely amazing.

We timed our trip to Sydney with New Year's Eve and planned to watch the world-famous fireworks at Sydney Harbour. Martina had sussed it all out beforehand and realised that alcohol would be prohibited in the area and everyone would be searched as they went through. Alcohol would cost a fortune if we brought it from the stands, so we came up with a cunning plan and tied a box of wine underneath my wheelchair and hoped for the best! As we had suspected, nobody took any notice of innocent old me and we had a merry night, welcoming in the New Year.

Although we had an absolute brilliant holiday, one thing was constantly on my mind - my placement year. It hung over me like a black cloud and I worried about my future. If I couldn't even find a placement for a year, what were my chances of finding full-time employment once I graduated? One night during our holiday, the stress all got too much and while chatting to Martina, I just broke down in tears. I realised then how stressed I'd been. I began to wonder if I should just give up, do my final year and then worry about finding a job. But I'd never been a quitter and it just didn't sit right with me. My peers were all sorted and I was still applying for placements, which were by now, dwindling. My exams were fast approaching and I was in danger of spreading myself far too thinly. But sharing my concerns with Martina helped and I knew, one way or another, I'd find a placement.

Refreshed and more determined than ever, I returned to Brookes to refocus my placement search. As a final resort, I decided to visit the University's Careers Centre. Strictly speaking, it wasn't their domain to find sandwich placements and there wasn't much they could do that I hadn't tried, but they saw my desperation and agreed to try and help me. A lady called Marie decided she'd try cold calling a few local councils to see if they had any suitable opportunities that would meet the placement requirements. Our determination paid off. Reading Borough Council were working in partnership with Scope to set up a project to support disabled people into work and they needed a project assistant. How amazing was that after my recent experience?

There were funding issues, as is always the case with publically funded projects, but they were very keen to meet me. I was asked to meet the team in Reading for what they had stressed would be a fairly informal interview. My career advisor and friend, Sue, had offered to come with me in support, given my past interview experience with the company in Oxford. But when we arrived in Reading, I was feeling confident, so Sue agreed to meet me after the interview.

It was a hot day and I was led into a small interview room. There were four people sat around the table – so much for the interview being informal. More like an interrogation! I was quickly reassured; they had all seen my CV and liked what they saw. They were particularly amused and impressed by my example of determination – taking and failing my driving test seven times. Although I still hadn't secured a full driving licence, it at least demonstrated commitment and perseverance if nothing else!

The interview was more of a discussion as the team outlined the project to me and what my role would be. As project assistant, I would be playing a key role in developing and promoting the project, which didn't yet have a name. I would be developing marketing materials, organising promotional events and helping to get a website up and running. I was going to be a busy girl and the way everyone was talking, the job was mine!

I can't tell you how good it felt to have finally secured my first real job. I don't think anybody had ever really considered the possibility of me working and supporting myself. And now it was happening – I was firmly in the real world and it felt brilliant! I couldn't wait to tell my folks and boyfriend at the time, Dean. I went to meet Sue as agreed and she was almost as thrilled as I was. In true Irish style, we found the nearest Irish pub to toast my success!

It was probably the first time I'd made a major decision without consulting anyone. I was going where the work was and that meant moving to Reading. It was daunting – I'd found a job and now I had to find somewhere to live. That would be no easy task.

For the first six weeks of my contract, until I found accommodation in Reading, I commuted from Oxford for three days a week and worked remotely in my Halls of Residence for two days. I was exhausted and yet it felt brilliant – I was just like anyone else commuting to work and beginning to pay my way in the world.

Chapter 17
Commuting hell

As I said, I felt like any other person commuting to work and I embraced it. But there was one thing I had to contend with which other commuters didn't – the lazy, ignorant bus drivers. No, I'm not going to mince my words here! Each morning, I'd wait at the bus stop and watch the driver's face as they approached. It didn't seem to matter which driver it was, the look I received was always the same: dread and annoyance. Why? Because the driver couldn't be bothered to get out of his seat to put the ramp out for me. All of the buses had the ramps and had to have them by law. But on these particular buses, they were fold up ramps which were kept in a box just behind the driver's cab. Their reluctance to get the ramps out and let me on to the bus was pure and simple laziness. And perhaps fear that if, God forbid, they took the time to get the ramp out (all of a minute or so) their bus might end up being late.

Some mornings, the driver (and as I said, they were all as bad) made an excuse and refused to put me on to the bus. They didn't give any thought as to whether their bad attitude would make me late for work. Other mornings, I was made to feel like a nuisance and it was embarrassing getting on to the bus in front of the other passengers.

As the summer progressed, I began to dread my commute to work and my initial enthusiasm had disappeared. Commuting to work was all the more stressful because of some ignorant, selfish jobs-worth idiots. Told you I wouldn't mince my words! The situation was starting to get me down when my big sis, Martina, came to visit me.

I was excited to tell Martina all about my new job – she'd known about my struggle to secure a placement and as always, had been very supportive. But I also told her about my daily battle with the bus drivers and the next day, she was able to witness the struggle I encountered each day. We were going into town and as the bus approached us, I got the usual 'look'. Now I had a companion, the driver knew he'd have to actually comply with the law and provide the ramp. But boy did he make it crystal clear what an inconvenience it was. He huffed and puffed, pulled faces and then dumped the ramp down in front of me.

I was getting used to this kind of attitude and aggression, but Martina was absolutely furious! Once I was on board, she decided to approach the driver and ask him if he had a problem with doing his job. He retorted that his job was to drive a bus, but Martina had big news for him. His job was not to just simply drive a bus, it was to transport passengers and to that end, he was required to do whatever was required to enable passengers to access the bus. I couldn't have put it better myself and I was so proud of my big sister. She took his badge number and when we got off the bus, we noted the bus details. I'd finally had enough and Martina's stand had inspired me to make a formal complaint.

By the time I got a reply, I had moved down to Reading, but the bus company sent me a profuse apology and £30 in vouchers to use.

Thinking about it now, it's not like me to just put up with things for so long, but I think I was worried about making a complaint while I still relied on the buses. I knew that they'd realise it was me and I didn't want to make the experience any worse than it was.

Eventually, I found a lovely two bedroom apartment in the centre of Reading and thankfully, no longer had to rely on the buses. I settled in at work and absolutely loved my job. Helping people who were in the same situation as I had been gave me a huge amount of satisfaction. Within weeks of starting my placement, I was told that an Away-day was being organised in the Isle of Wight in order to plan out one of the projects and I would be required to go. While I was excited, I was also nervous. I didn't yet know anybody in the team and I knew even less about the project. This could be disastrous!

One of my line managers was also going, so the pressure was on to prove to him that I was capable. We spent most of the time working in groups and despite my inexperience, I was able to contribute to the discussion and even come up with some ideas. With my confidence growing, I volunteered to feed back our ideas to the rest of group. My nervousness disappeared and I was delighted when everyone was able to understand me and some of my ideas were incorporated into the project plan.

My line manager was a straight talking, no nonsense man and he later took me aside to congratulate me on my performance, saying it 'took balls' to throw myself in at the deep end like I had. He was impressed with my can-do attitude and I knew that I'd made a good impression. My career was off to a flying start!

Chapter 18
Kindness of strangers

Dean and I were still maintaining a long distance relationship, but it was becoming increasingly difficult. He came to see me whenever he could and, whenever possible, I got the coach down to Southend-on-Sea for a couple of days. But the visits were infrequent and the strain of trying to maintain the relationship began to show.

We continued to talk about a long-term future together when I graduated, but as our relationship progressed it became evident that our visions for that future were very different. Although it took me a long time to see it, we weren't the best match. I had my future mapped out in my head - finish my degree, secure a good job and then settle down to marriage and kids, perhaps start my own business. Things were different for Dean and I knew he was anxious for me to complete my degree and move down to be with him in Southend. But that was a long way from my home and family in Ireland and I had a lot to achieve before settling down. We argued about almost every aspect of life – where we'd live, how many kids we'd have and how we would support ourselves.

Getting to university had been my dream and I was very focused on my degree and although we continued to see each other whenever we could, it was becoming clear that Dean and I were drifting apart. I was working so hard to get my degree and Dean had a group of friends that I wasn't apart of and I think we both felt isolated from each other's lives. A long distance relationship is difficult at the best of times, but when you add to that both parties having disabilities and me trying to focus on my degree and build a proper career, it was never going to work. Neither of us could drive and neither of us had much money to spend on travelling, so we very rarely saw each other. Although we spoke to each other every day and spent hours on the phone, looking back on it now, I realise it wasn't a real relationship and we both deserved better.

So after five years together, Dean finally ended our relationship for good. It was Easter Monday 2005 when Dean phoned me and I knew from his voice that something wasn't right. Over the years, we'd had several break-ups and each time it happened, I was devastated. As Dean explained that he wanted to break up again, I was convinced we'd be back together within a few days. But Dean insisted that this time it was for good and he turned out to be right. It absolutely broke my heart and it took me a long time to rebuild my confidence. I was convinced I'd never find anyone to share my life with and that scared me. I just couldn't see anyone accepting me for who I was, unless they had a disability themselves and understood me. Dean had been a brilliant companion as he had been able to relate to my strengths, weaknesses and challenges. He'd been in my life for five and a half years, had been my best friend and like most people would, I struggled with our break-up. As I said, we'd had several temporary splits over the years and I was convinced that with time, we'd once again get back together.

But as the days turned to weeks and the weeks into months, my phone remained silent and I slowly realised that this time, Dean wasn't coming back and I felt so alone. I'd been just sixteen when I'd met Dean and now I suddenly felt a bubble had burst and I had to find my own way. But I hadn't just lost Dean. I'd been quite close to his Mum and over the years, she'd been a good friend to me and now, understandably, she had to be loyal to Dean, so she too severed all contact with me. I was truly heartbroken and I don't think I've ever felt so alone.

But somehow, I had to pull myself together for the sake of completing my work placement and my degree. In a few months' time, I'd be returning to Oxford to face the final year of my degree, but without Dean's support and encouragement, I knew it would be tough – particularly as I'd also be missing the new friends that I'd made in Reading. I was utterly determined to pick myself up, even if my confidence was in tatters.

But worse was to come once I'd returned to Oxford. My Nan became very ill and was hospitalised. As well as trying to focus on my exams and dissertation, I spent most weekends in Birmingham visiting Nan. It was clear that she was nearing the end of her life and as a family, we were devastated. She finally passed away on 26 November – on what would have been my sixth anniversary with Dean. I'd been dreading the day for weeks, wondering what I'd do to distract myself, but now I was heartbroken for a very different reason. I spent the next few days in a daze – I hardly slept at night. As daft as it might sound, I was scared that I'd dream about Nan. Being in my final year, I couldn't afford to miss too much work, so despite the lack of sleep, I was still going to my lectures.

I was like a zombie and one afternoon, I realised I'd dozed off, only to be woken by the phone. I'd expected it to be Mum, confirming the funeral arrangements and I was caught completely off guard when I heard Dean's voice. We hadn't spoken in the eight months since we'd split up, but he'd heard about Nan and wanted to sympathise. It was a kind gesture and though I was still hurting, it paved the way for us to become friends again. I was starting to accept that Dean had moved on, but it was great to have his friendship at such a difficult time.

Despite the heartache, I don't regret the time that I spent with Dean. It taught me so much about myself and I grew up a lot in those five years. Although we've had our ups and down since, we're now Facebook friends and there's no longer any animosity between us. But he finds it funny that my husband's name is Dean!

Despite the heartache of splitting with Dean, I'd successfully completed my one year placement in Reading and the project which I'd helped get off the ground was starting to flourish. When I'd started my placement, it was really just an idea. The project didn't even have a name and we had no clients, although we knew there were plenty of people who needed our support. We were based in council offices which didn't make us very accessible. There was a lot of work to be done in order to get the project off the ground and I threw myself into it.

Twelve months on and we were starting to make a difference to the lives of disabled people who were looking for employment. It was clear that the support we offered was desperately needed and valued, not just by individuals themselves, but by other support organisations who couldn't offer the same level of support. On a personal level, I was in my element! I was all too aware of how difficult it was to secure employment when faced with a disability and now I was helping people who were in the exact same position that I had been just 12 months earlier. I was also earning a living and living completely independently for the first time ever.

I knew that all too soon, I'd have to return to Oxford to complete the final year of my degree. I was so proud of what I'd helped to achieve in Reading and I knew the project had the potential to grow beyond its initial first year of funding and I desperately wanted to be a part of that. After some discussion with my bosses, it was evident that they would welcome my return once I had graduated. As Scope was still a main stakeholder in the project, I was asked to apply for their Graduate Recruitment Scheme, which was specifically for disabled graduates. If successful, Scope would place me back on the project, this time as a junior manager.

I worked hard on my application form and after a few months, I was invited to London for an interview and Assessment Centre. Although I'd obviously had interviews before, I'd never done an Assessment Centre before and I had no idea what to expect. I was petrified! Given my previous interview experience, Sue offered to accompany me and it was an offer that I couldn't refuse.

As we travelled down to London on the train, Sue

put me through my paces. She threw question after question at me and we'd perfect the answers until they were ingrained on my memory. We went through what I might expect from the Assessment Centre and how I might respond to any tricky questions. Although this graduate programme was specifically aimed at disabled graduates, my previous interview for the Oxford marketing company was playing on my mind and I wanted to ensure that as well as promoting my strengths, I could combat any doubts they might have about my disability. I was a bag of nerves and as we pulled into Paddington, I was just concentrating on keeping calm. As we had to wait for assistance, we let our fellow passengers disembark first. I was overwhelmed as one by one, they wished me good luck for the interview! The carriage had been fairly quiet and they must have heard me practising, I must have driven them mad with all the repetition, but here they were, wishing me the best. I was very touched and it gave me the extra confidence boost that I so desperately needed.

Sue and I made our way to Lehman Brothers in Canary Wharf, where the interviews were being held. Being in such a formal, corporate environment was exciting, but it did nothing to calm my nerves! I was so grateful that Sue was there to support me and though I knew she couldn't go through the process for me, her coaching and mentoring got me through the day.

Two days prior to the interview, I'd been asked to prepare a presentation and delivering it to the panel was my first task of the day. As I've mentioned, I always get nervous when talking to people I don't know and worry that they won't be able to understand what I'm saying. So whenever I give a presentation now, I always start by saying that if anyone can't understand me, they should just let me know as I don't mind repeating myself. And I really don't, as one of my pet hates is when people just pretend that they are getting it when it's clear to me that they can't understand a word – I can always tell! As I got started, my confidence grew and by the end of the presentation, I felt fairly happy with my performance and having watched from the corner of the room, Sue reassured me that it had gone down well.

It was a tiring day and having completed a one-to-one interview and an in-tray exercise, it was time for a group exercise which would be observed by the panel of interviewers. I knew what they would be looking for – someone with leadership and conflict resolution skills. But as the exercise began, I started to panic. We were each given a 'role' to play and some listed points which we were required to get across in the discussion, but we weren't permitted to discuss the information that we'd been given with the other participants. As the conversation progressed, I realised that the exercise wasn't going to be as easy as I'd hoped and I soon found myself backed into a corner which I couldn't get out of without revealing too much to the others. I didn't know what to do so I decided to raise my hand and ask for clarification from the panel. I felt an idiot, but either way, I'd messed up the exercise. Or so I thought.

I got through the rest of the exercise, but after such a promising day, I was convinced I'd failed by asking for clarification and I couldn't stop beating myself up about it. Much to my surprise, a few days later I took a call from one of the interviewers who informed me that they'd been very impressed by my performance and I'd been offered a place on the programme! Far from letting myself down, I'd demonstrated confidence and initiative by asking for clarification. The interviewers knew they'd put me in a tricky situation, but they were delighted with the way I'd handled it! I was over the moon as I phoned to tell Sue the good news and thank her for all her support.

I was invited to an open day to meet all of the employers who were signed up to the Graduate Scheme, but I didn't see the point in going. I knew that there was a job in Reading with my name on it and I couldn't wait to get back to it. All I had to do was complete my final year at Brookes.

That final year of university was probably my best. I was getting over my split with Dean and getting used to only having myself to think about. My placement year in Reading had helped me to grow up and I was excited about the future because it was *my* future – I decided where it would take me and I no longer had the pressure to settle down in a town I didn't know, miles from any of my friends or family. (Although it's ironic, as that's almost exactly what I did!)

Before my placement year, university had been a chore – something to endure and survive, rather than enjoy. I'd constantly felt isolated and insecure – everyone on my course had their group of friends and I never felt like I fitted in. Always on the outside, looking in – that's how I felt. My placement year had been very different – I'd made some good friends through work and I always felt wanted and included. I'd also lived completely independently for the first time and so when the end of my placement approached, I began to dread my return to Oxford.

I need not have worried: my time in Reading had given me so much more confidence and that stood me in good stead for my final year. Within weeks of returning, I was paired with a guy called Stepan to work on a joint assignment and gradually, I got to know him and his housemates. They lived around the corner from my Halls of Residence and 'number 22', as we referred to their place, became my second home. I'd be there at least a few nights each week and even though we had finished our assignment, we were both working hard on our dissertations and it was great to have someone who understood the pressure I was under. I finally felt relaxed and at ease – this was how university should be and having such good people around me helped me further in getting over my split with Dean. My new friends, Stepan, Mark and Margaret, gave me the support and encouragement that had once come from him.

Although they were not always a good influence. Up until that point, I hardly ever touched alcohol (and if you believe that, then as the Irish would say, you're a right eejit!) I was passing number 22 one day to go shopping and Margaret was outside. She had decided to have an afternoon off her studies and was going to settle down in front of the TV. She convinced me to join her (my arm was really twisted. . .) and by the end of the evening, we'd polished off two bottles of red wine! How I ever passed my final year and completed my dissertation, I'll never know, but that was definitely the best year of my time in Oxford, even though another unexplained complaint started during that final year.

Out of nowhere, my left arm started going very stiff and heavy. I couldn't get it to do what I wanted it to do and just as when my speech had nose-dived, I really didn't understand what was happening. It was my final year and though I was working hard and naturally a little stressed, I was looking after myself and felt in control of my workload.

My arm was continually heavy and I often had to use my right hand to lift it or else just manage one handed. It was tough and unexplained, so I went to visit my GP who, not knowing much about CP, referred me to the local hospital. Before any treatment could be considered, I was told that I'd need an MRI Scan just to rule out anything nasty that might be causing this deterioration in my otherwise predictable condition.

Remembering my childhood experiences of MRI scans, I was petrified. I was told that although the hospital would be unwilling to give me a general anaesthetic for such a simple procedure, they would offer me sedation. Though this eased my fears somewhat, I was still dreading the scan and worrying about what it might reveal. Nonetheless, I wanted the problem dealt with, so I kept the appointment. As is often the case, I'd built things up so much in my head, getting myself into a right state and the reality wasn't half as bad. The sedation really relaxed me and I was even able to listen to some music while the scan was being done and it was over before I knew it.

But once again, the scan failed to show anything unusual and so the stiffness in my arm went unexplained, but not untreated. I was told that they could inject Botox directly into the muscles which would help to relax them and ease my discomfort. I'd always thought Botox was for vain celebrities with more money than sense and I was quite surprised to learn that it could help my condition. The consultant also noticed the constant movement in my head, what I refer to as the nodding dog effect, and said I could also have injections into my neck to help control the movements. But I wasn't keen on that, especially as the movement doesn't bother me much and with some effort, can be controlled. I just wanted to be able to use my arm normally again, so it was agreed that I'd have the injections every three months and eventually, I was told, the stiffness would correct itself.

   I got a bit of a kick out of telling friends that I was having Botox - I'd watch for their reaction and then explain the *real* purpose of it! Like me, it surprised a lot of people that it could be used for the purposes of controlling a medical condition rather than for cosmetic reasons and it really did work. Almost immediately, it completely relaxed the muscles and my arm returned to that mystical state of *'normal'* again. In the past, I had taken medication to try and control spasms, but the injections were much more effective and preferable to taking pills every day. Besides, there was an added bonus in that my arm became wrinkle free!

Chapter 19
Sixty-one point three

So now I'd come to the end of yet another chapter in my life. After many stressful nights, many tears, dozens of assignments and exams, one dissertation and a couple of drunken nights in the Student Union, I'd finally completed my degree. My time in Oxford hadn't always been easy, but even without my final results, I had achieved so much and grown up a lot.

My fears about not been able to secure full-time employment had proved to be unfounded and I was looking forward to returning to Reading and carving out a new life for myself. As it happened, I'd also kept in touch with my old landlady who was thinking about selling the apartment which I'd rented during my placement year. It had been so convenient and accessible that it made sense for me to buy it rather than waste money renting. I liked Reading and I was happy to settle there, for a while anyway.

As I waited for the sale to go through and my start date in Reading to be confirmed, I returned to Birmingham for a few weeks. Despite all the exciting changes which were ahead of me, there was just one thing that I couldn't stop thinking about. My final results. I'd be more than happy with a 2:1 – as they say, a drinking man's degree! That had been my goal throughout the whole four years and the majority of my grades were consistent with a 2:1 but I doubted whether I'd make it. My results were going to be published online and I was staying with Mum and Dad in their house in Birmingham, but unfortunately, they didn't have the internet.

Results day had finally dawned and we went in search of an internet connection. I was a bundle of nerves and excitement as we drove to the local library. I could hardly log into the system, I was shaking so much. Dad had to help me navigate to the right page and then I glanced down: 61.3 percent. I thought that must relate to one of my exams. Then I looked again. No, that was definitely my overall percentage and it equalled a 2:1 Honours degree. By the skin of my teeth, I'd got my 2:1. Mum and Dad weren't sure what they were looking at and through tears, I told them I'd done it! The three of us just sat there, looking at the screen, double checking what it meant. I honestly couldn't believe it! Just to be sure, I even phoned the university and they confirmed my results.

As with my GCSE results, they couldn't wait to tell anyone who would listen. The library assistant was hovering near by and when she saw our tears, Mum was only too delighted to tell her that I'd just achieved a 2:1 honours degree!

To most people, their degree gets them onto the career ladder and helps them to secure a slightly better salary, though that isn't always the case. To me, it didn't matter what job I ended up with or how much I might earn. All that mattered was that I'd achieved my goal. A goal that so many people along the way thought was impossible for me to achieve. Like I said before, I'm not a told-you-so kind of person, not at all!

I'd only been in my new job for a few weeks when I had to take a day off, but my boss was more than happy to agree and even congratulated me. . . It was my graduation and I didn't intend to miss it!

The day started with a disaster. I'd booked myself in to have my hair done – only I didn't really know Reading that well and had just booked the first hairdresser that I came across in town. Big mistake! With just hours until my graduation, my hair looked like a frizzy bird's nest! When Mum and Dad arrived to pick me up, Mum took one look at me and asked if I'd even been to the hairdressers! I knew then that it was bad and Mum offered to wash out the 'curls' and redo it for me. With no time to spare I had very little choice, but to her credit, Mum salvaged the situation and when

I looked presentable again, we made our way to Oxford.

I was excited and nervous as we approached the university. As well as my family who had all travelled from Ireland, some of my friends were also coming to share my big day, including my ex, Dean. At that point, we were just about ready to be friends again and despite everything, he was proud of what I'd achieved and I was pleased that he wanted to share my special day.

After saying hello to everyone, it was time to get organised! While Mum tried to locate some hair grips to keep my cap in place, Dad came with me to get registered and collect my certificate (the one they give out during the ceremony isn't the real thing!) As I gave in my details, the lady informed me that I would be going up onto the stage twice and I was a bit confused. When we'd rehearsed things, nobody had mentioned going up twice. When I queried the reason why, the lady smiled and said that I'd been awarded a prize! I was absolutely gob-smacked. When the lady explained that it was in recognition of my achievements as a disabled student, Dad was absolutely thrilled! We wandered outside and decided to take a peek at my certificate. As I pulled it from the envelope, Dad's eyes welled up and he couldn't stop grinning. As the crowds buzzed around us, we knew we'd better move, but it was a wonderful moment which has been etched on my memory ever since.

The ceremony was a dream come true and to my relief, my cap remained firmly in place throughout, despite my head shaking! The university had made great efforts to ensure that I could enjoy the moment just like my peers by installing a ramp and positioning me in the best possible place. After receiving my degree, I wasn't quite sure when I would be called for the award of the prize: to be honest, I thought maybe there had been a mistake and I wouldn't be called up again. But towards the end of the ceremony, the Dean began speaking about a new award for disabled students and I knew I hadn't been dreaming. As I went to collect it, all I could hear were claps and cheers!

It was a wonderful day and I was thrilled to have achieved what I'd set out to. It had been a long four years and I'd had many difficult times, including splitting up with Dean after over five years together and losing my Nan as I was doing my finals. But I'd got there and I'd got so much more than just a degree. I'd got my independence and now I had secured a permanent, full-time management position and I had my own apartment.

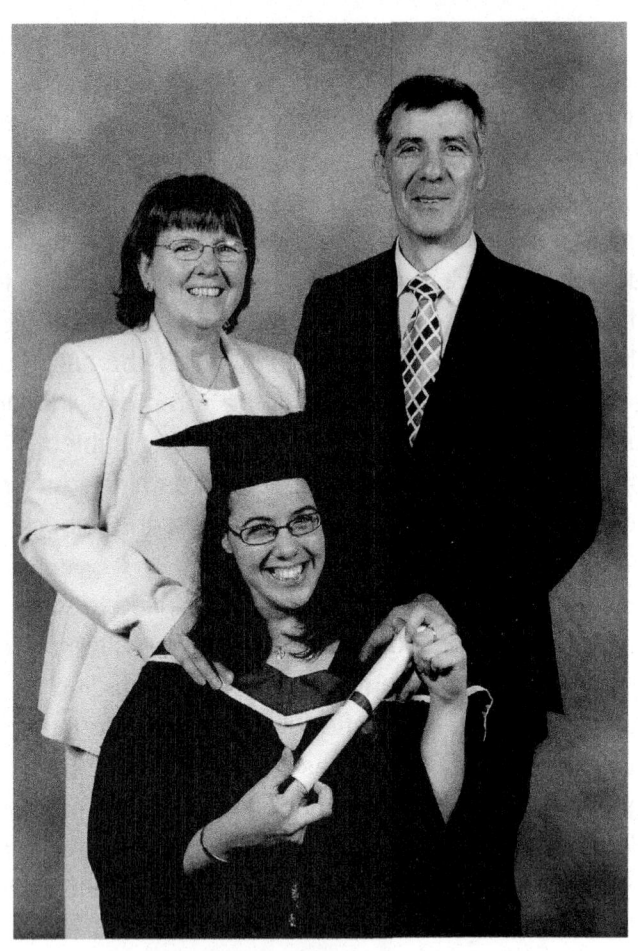

As well as a 2:1 Honours Degree, I won a prize in recognition of my achievements as a disabled student

Chapter 20
Me, myself and I

Moving back to Reading, into my own home, was a huge milestone for me. I was going to be living independently for the first time *ever.* In the past I'd always had flatmates around or carers on call, should I need them. But this time, it was just me, myself and I. As I picked up the keys for my first home, I was so excited, but also very anxious. I'd been working towards this for years and now, I finally had my independence.

As they had done several times before, Mum and Dad got me settled in my new pad, making sure the kitchen was well stocked and the flat was spotlessly clean before they left me. This time, as Mum and Dad pulled away, I was full of excitement. My experiences at Hereward and then at university, had given me so much confidence and I knew I'd be just fine. It would be nice to have my own space, but I still couldn't believe that the flat was mine. Not only did I own my own home, I had a full-time job and would be supporting myself completely. Whoever would have believed it? I certainly never dared to believe that I'd achieve quite so much by the age of twenty-three. That first night, completely by myself, was weird. I'd locked the door but every little noise troubled me until I got used to living alone.

But living alone presented many other challenges. Although I knew how to cook a limited menu, it was physically quite difficult to prepare a proper meal. Whenever I did attempt it, I was always very hesitant in case I burned myself or cut a finger. Although it was reassuring to know that the local hospital was just across the road! More often than not, in those early days of living alone, I relied mostly on microwavable meals or takeaways. It was far from a healthy diet, but it was easier and safer for me to do that than try and cook for myself, particularly after a long day at work when I was tired.

I also had another predicament - getting the food from the kitchen into the lounge, where the dining table was. Simply carrying it through wasn't an option, as most of it would end up on the floor! Instead, I'd put my plate on the kitchen floor, get down on my hands and knees and slide my plate along the floor until I got into the lounge. I'd then go back and get my cutlery. It was a slow process but it was the only way that I could guarantee keeping a decent amount of food on the plate! I did the same with my washing - yank it out of the washing machine and push and pull the pile of clothes along the floor, until I reached the clothes horse which was in the bathroom. I'd then sit on the edge of the bath and hang it all up. It took me ages, but at least I was doing it myself and that felt good.

When I was little, I was assessed by a doctor who observed that I'd often solve a problem, without even realising that there was one to solve. For example, knowing that I couldn't lift a drink without spilling it, I'd go down to the cup rather than trying to lift it to my mouth and I did it without even realising what I was doing. I'd just find the best way for me to do things and that ability has stayed with me. There aren't many things that will beat me, because I value my independence so much.

But even so, even I had to accept that there were some things that I simply couldn't do and I'd have to wait until someone visited to ask for help. Trying to change my bed by myself was a nightmare and could take me all afternoon! I'd get into such a flap and it just frustrated me. Anne, a friend from work, was brilliant and whenever she came, she would help me to change it and often take me shopping. Although I could carry a decent amount of shopping on the back of my wheelchair, it was difficult to carry the bulky items and I was incredibly grateful to Anne for those shopping trips. It could be annoying when a light bulb went and I had no way of changing it myself. As I got to know some of the neighbours, I felt more comfortable asking them for the odd favour. As they lived upstairs, I'd leave my front door open and try to catch them as they came in from work.

The neighbours weren't the only ones I had to try to catch though. It had been a very long day at work and I was looking forward to getting home and settling down in front of the TV. But as I opened my front door, something caught my eye. At first, I wasn't sure what it was, but then it appeared again. A mouse was running around my flat! I let out such a scream, I'm surprised none of the neighbours heard me. I couldn't believe it, but I didn't have a clue what to do. The mouse was so quick, I didn't stand a chance of catching it, so once again, I waited for my neighbour from upstairs to come home. I felt like such a weak girl asking him to help me, but I just couldn't face sorting this out on my own! We discovered the mice were getting in through a broken vent by my kitchen and as it was so late, there was little I could do until the morning. I didn't get much sleep that night, I can tell you! With the help of Pest Control and some mouse traps, I eventually got rid of my little visitors. It wasn't pleasant having to dispose of the debris and it would have been handy to have someone around then!

Despite these difficulties, I loved living on my own. The freedom felt great and I loved working and being able to look after myself. Securing my first full-time, permanent job was a major achievement. I got the impression when I was younger that nobody really expected me to be capable of working and even if I was, it would be very difficult for me to get an employer to see beyond my disability. But I didn't want to fit the stereotypical view of disabled people – unable or unwilling to work and happy to have the state support them. That wasn't me and I hadn't been brought up that way. I'd watched Mum and Dad work their fingers to the bone, seven days a week and eventually they'd been rewarded and we had a nice car and some good holidays. I wanted a good job and I wanted to pay my way in life, just as my parents had.

When I decided to accept the graduate post in Reading, I had been promised a role as a junior manager and the intention was to train me up to take on more responsibility. I was thrilled and being such a small organisation, I had a real opportunity to make a difference. Initially my role involved promoting the organisation, organising events to provide clients with work experience opportunities and assisting with the general running of the project.

One of our main aims was to educate employers about the benefits of employing a diverse workforce. After my previous experience, I was passionate about working with employers and helping them to recognise that disabled people had a lot to offer. To this end, I was heavily involved in organising promotional events which we called, quite simply, 'Hotel Days'. The idea was that we'd take over a local hotel for the day, staff it with our clients and then prepare and serve lunch to invited local employers and dignitaries. I loved these events as they always gave our clients a much needed confidence boost and sometimes resulted in them securing further work experience or even paid work. The media always gave us good coverage and I got such a buzz from seeing the event come together, often after months of planning and hard work. It was particularly rewarding to see clients undertaking work experience, often for the first time, realising that despite their impairments they were capable of contributing to society.

As I said before, my ultimate motivation was to help people who were in a similar situation to the one I had been in; I knew how frustrating it was for people to ignore my skills and judge my capabilities purely on the basis of my disability. Scope, a national disability charity, were a major partner in our project and were aware of my previous challenges trying to secure employment. I was excited as well as extremely honoured when they asked me to front one of their national campaigns which would raise awareness of the discrimination which disabled people face *and* also raise money which Scope would use to fund their employment programme. My struggle to find employment and my subsequent success would form a case study which would be sent to Scope's supporters across the country. I worked with Scope's marketing team on getting the case study just right and I was delighted with the results. I only hoped that it would help make a difference to some disabled people who were facing the same struggles that I had. A few months later, Scope let me know that the campaign had raised over £50,000! I was over the moon that I'd been part of it.

But as hard as I worked to change attitudes towards disabled people, the discrimination that existed was still all too evident. I remember answering a phone call one day from a potential new client who was looking for some support to find a job. He was quite angry as he questioned why, 'someone with cerebral palsy' could get a job while he remained unemployed. I was flabbergasted by his attitude, particularly as he was expecting me to help him! I was fuming as I ended the call and told my colleagues what he had said. The guy never bothered making contact again, such was his disgust that someone with CP was actually able to get a job: Heaven forbid, that they might perhaps help him get one too!

On another occasion, my manager and I had gone out to a meeting and had decided to get a taxi back to the office. I was well used to bad attitudes from taxi drivers in Reading - many of whom claimed that they couldn't carry wheelchairs, even though they are required by law to carry ramps. Most of them just couldn't be bothered - my money clearly wasn't good enough for them. On this occasion, the driver took us, but treated me like I was dumb and refused to talk to me, instead directing everything to my manager. By the time we got to the office, I was fuming and decided to take my revenge. I paid the £15 fare all in small change and made him wait while I counted it all out!

It was hard work and frustrating at times but I loved my job and always gave 100% commitment. I was often the first in and the last to leave, but I didn't care – I believed in our cause and that kept me going. Each and every Friday evening, I'd be so tired that I could barely speak and loved my Saturday mornings in bed! My commitment was rewarded when I was nominated for the Sue Ryder 'Woman of Achievement' award in 2007 by my manager, as well as by the overall project manager at Reading Borough Council. I was both touched and thrilled that my work was making such a difference and was being recognised. As part of the nominations, I was featured in the local paper and as a team we attended the Awards Ceremony in Henley-on-Thames. Although I didn't win, we all had a lovely evening and if nothing else, it helped to raise the profile of our project locally.

Chapter 21

Free-wheeling

Throughout my childhood, my parents fought many battles on my behalf and as you have seen, they were pretty successful. They fought tooth and nail for what was right for me and subsequently taught me that you should be prepared to fight for what you need and to expect to win. But there is one fight I have not yet won and it affects many more people than just me: our daily struggle against the general ignorance and apathy towards disability.

Although I can walk short distances, my electric wheelchair and my four wheels are, effectively, my legs. So whenever something goes wrong with it, it's almost as if I've broken a leg: my chair is the key to my independence, without it I can't go anywhere or do anything by myself. That's a bit of a problem when you're trying to hold down a full-time job with management responsibilities. My chair had been provided by the NHS who appointed contractors to oversee the maintenance and repair of all their wheelchairs. Whenever something went wrong, I had to contact the appointed contractor. Unfortunately, they were rarely up to the job.

It was coming up to Christmas and just like everyone else, I had a lot to do and many places to go! Of all the times for my wheelchair to go, now was definitely not a good time. It was never easy to get it repaired at the best of times, so I was dreading the inevitable battle which lay ahead. I phoned them and explained that my chair wasn't working, I was at home but was due at work and could someone please come out as soon as possible? I was told an engineer could visit, 'sometime tomorrow'. There was very little I could do except to phone my manager and explain my predicament. I had no choice but to take a day off work and wait. But when the engineer finally arrived the next day, it wasn't good news. He couldn't fix it and would have to take it back to the workshop for three days! THREE DAYS? What was I supposed to do in the mean time? I'd be completely confined to the apartment, unless I paid out for taxis and even then, I couldn't get around easily in my manual wheelchair. I asked if there was a spare chair which could be loaned to me while mine was being repaired, but I was simply told they didn't have any available and that was that.

At the time, I lived alone, I was working full-time and I felt that it was unacceptable to leave me with no means of getting around. So I decided to phone the contractor again to try and make them understand my situation. I got the impression that most of their clients attended day care centre and had care support and therefore didn't totally rely on their electric wheelchairs as I did.

Again, the response I got from the receptionist was far from helpful as she told me to 'go have a cup of tea and calm down.' Calm down? I wondered how calm she would be if she couldn't leave her house, through no fault of her own and had to explain to her employers why she couldn't make it into work. At the time, I was managing a difficult staff member who thought nothing of ringing in sick on a weekly basis with some lame excuse or other. I was trying to reduce her absences and set a good example, but at the moment I couldn't make it into work myself.

On that particular occasion, those three days turned into well over a week and eventually the engineer realised that the chair was beyond repair and I would need a new one. I could hardly believe it; they'd left me a week without any mobility, only to tell me that they were putting the chair on the scrapheap!

Whenever I had needed a wheelchair in the past, my needs had been carefully assessed and then I had been provided with the most appropriate wheelchair. However, on this occasion, I was told that the wheelchair department only had one chair available which was eight years old. It was very basic and offered very little support for my back, which was often in bits. I was offered a few cushions and more or less told to take it or leave it. It was more of an indoor chair than an outdoor chair and I knew it wasn't up to my level of usage, but I had little choice.

This kind of approach goes back to the Medical Model of Disability which had been the torment of my early life – people see a 'problem' to be solved and so they solve it. I needed an electric chair and they gave me one. But there's no consideration for the individual at the centre of it. They didn't concern themselves with what I actually needed the chair to do, because they assumed all their clients were the same – not working and attending a day care facility where help was always on hand.

That's why I found dealing with the contractor so difficult. I was never treated as an individual and my needs were never fully met. I was one of hundreds and another box to tick, another cheque to claim. Each phone call was a battle and I was always aware that they didn't really care whether or not I made it to work. And they thought a cup of tea would calm me down? It wouldn't come close, I don't even drink tea!

It never took long for the chair to start playing up again and this time, it had been acting up for weeks and each time the engineer came out, he reckoned it was fixed; within days, it would start cutting out again – sometimes in the middle of the road. I knew the chair wasn't right and I knew I was vulnerable – the chair might just give up and I could end up stranded on a main road somewhere. I was at work one day when the wheelchair started its tricks once again. It was really getting to me down now and I was seriously worried about it dying altogether. Even though the chair was still mobile (just), I rang the contractor and explained that the chair was dodgy and intermittent and as I was at work, I was concerned about getting home safely. I was told that the engineer didn't have any free slots for three days.

The receptionist really didn't understand the seriousness of the situation and after so many call outs, I was on the verge of losing my patience. I took a long, deep breath and asked how she expected me to get home safely that evening. Her response was deadly serious: 'Can't you free-wheel it home?' It took me a minute to process what she had said and I almost asked her to repeat herself, just to be sure that I'd heard correctly. Maybe I had wax in my ears? But no, I'd heard her alright and my blood was absolutely boiling. I had to make my explanation to her crystal clear this time:

'If I was capable of free-wheeling an electric wheelchair home, I wouldn't require the wheelchair in the first place, would I?' I said this slowly, just to ensure she'd understand, but I knew there was no point talking to her and so, shaking with anger, I asked to talk to her manager. She really was in the wrong job making statements like that. As I waited to be transferred to her manager, I was still gobsmacked. It was like telling someone with a broken leg to run a marathon and by this point, I was fuming.

After being put on hold, the receptionist eventually came back to me and said that the engineer would call to me later that day. However, my afternoon went from bad to worse when the engineer finally arrived. He took the chair to his van and must have been there for almost half an hour. But as my manager and I watched from the window, it was clear that he didn't have a clue how to fix it.

Eventually, he pushed the chair back to our office and announced that the chair was now worse that when he'd arrived. Whereas before, it had been intermittent but mobile, it now wasn't mobile at all. It was dead. The engineer announced that he didn't have the parts to fix it and casually said that he would return tomorrow. But where did that leave me? I was now stranded at work and when I pointed this out, the engineer shrugged his shoulders and told me it wasn't his responsibility to get me home safely. UNBELIEVABLE.

By this time, I was absolutely furious. The problems with my chair had been ongoing for weeks now and I had been scared to venture anywhere, other than work, just in case it cut out. The wheelchair service, if you can call it a service, had absolutely no clue about anything and didn't seem to care. Well, I wasn't about to let the engineer leave with no consequence, so I asked him to wait while I phoned his office – again. By now the phone number was engraved on my memory.

When the phone was answered, I took a deep sigh. It was the receptionist I'd dealt with earlier. I wasn't in the mood for this. Shaking with anger and pure frustration, I explained that not only had the engineer now broken my chair completely, he was now quite happy to leave me with no regard for how I would get home. After the fiasco earlier, I was stupidly expecting profuse apologies. But no. Her response was, 'Can't your carer take you home?'

The tears finally fell as I explained that no, my 'carer' couldn't take me home, I was at work, not a day care centre and I didn't have a carer. I can't describe how utterly frustrated and deflated I felt. Just because I was disabled, this woman had made the wild assumptions that a) I attended a day care facility and b) that I had a carer.

My manager was luckily still in the office and seeing my frustration, she took the phone from me and said that she would take me home. She was as shocked as I was at how I was being treated. I began thinking about the clients that I represented in my work, many of whom were also disabled and much more vulnerable than me. I knew that they faced similar challenges and felt it was only right that I should fight the injustice, not just for myself but for others that were less capable of making a stand. I've always been fortunate that Mum and Dad gave me the confidence to fight and demand better. This wasn't just about how the company had treated me – it was about other vulnerable people, who were just putting up with the same treatment because they weren't able to fight for better.

So the next day, I again phoned the contractor manager to make a formal complaint to the manager. Although he apologised and offered to pay some travel expenses, he wouldn't accept that his engineer (I use the term loosely) was at fault, firstly for breaking the chair and then failing to ensure that I got home safely. I was told that their contract was to service and repair wheelchairs and that was as far as their responsibilities went. He even had the audacity to quote the contract at me!

After months and even years of putting up with similar experiences, I decided enough was enough and bought a brand new wheelchair privately. It was much more supportive, faster and very comfortable. And there was a reliable call-out service who would respond quickly in the event of any problems. But I couldn't just walk away and let the wheelchair service get away with treating their clients as they did. As I said, it wasn't just about me. I wanted to make a difference for other people who were much more vulnerable than me. It was clear that the manager didn't see any need for changes, so rather than bang my head against a brick wall, I wrote to my local MP. I explained everything that had happened over the past few months and included all the comments made to me, which clearly demonstrated a huge lack of disability awareness.

My MP, Rob Wilson, promised to look into it on my behalf and within weeks, I had an appointment to go and meet the head of the NHS wheelchair department at the hospital. They wanted to offer me a new wheelchair. But it was too late for that – I'd already placed an order for a much more reliable and whizzy wheelchair. But I still wanted to attend the appointment as it gave me the perfect opportunity to tell the manager exactly what was going on in the company which he had commissioned and he seemed genuinely shocked by what I had to say.

As it turned out, the company were only supposed to make three call-outs for the same problem before reporting it to the hospital and referring the client for a wheelchair review. The hospital manager said that as a result of my complaint, they had invested in two new wheelchairs which would be loaned out to clients while their wheelchairs were repaired. It was progress, but it still relied on the engineers actually getting to the client – without them having to wait three days! Although I still wasn't satisfied that the needs of clients were being put first, I felt I had made my point and had put wheels in motion for change – excuse the pun!

A few days later, I heard that the wheelchair repair company had lost their contract and another provider was taking over with almost immediate effect. I don't know if my complaint had influenced that decision, but it didn't matter, I was absolutely delighted! It was a small victory for common sense, but I am afraid the fight to educate the general public that disabled people have feelings, rights and value will go on for many years yet. That challenge has led me to become professionally involved, but more of that later!

Chapter 22
All dolled up

When I was a young girl, Mum used to love dressing me up and my wardrobe was full of pretty dresses and my hair was always done nicely, normally in bunches or a French plait. I think I was Mum's little doll but I never complained. It was fun getting dressed up. Having two big sisters, I used to watch them getting ready for nights out, doing their hair, carefully applying their make-up, filing and then painting their nails. All the time, I wished that one day, I would perhaps be able to do the same thing.

But these days, I'm not really a girly girl, partly because it's so difficult for me to do things myself. My dexterity limits what I'm able to do with my hair and if I ever attempted to put on make-up, I was almost guaranteed to end up looking like a clown. It was as I grew into a teenager, that these things became more apparent and I knew things were different for me, compared to other girls.

Most of the girls at school took great pride in their appearance, often breaking the school rules on make-up and uniform. As I hit puberty, I started comparing myself to the other girls and I hated it. Even if Mum had allowed it, I wasn't able to put on make-up and I certainly wasn't able to shave my legs. I have quite thick, dark hair, so my hairy legs were extremely noticeable and it really bugged me. I always wore a skirt and socks to school as we weren't allowed to wear trousers so it was impossible to try and hide it. It was embarrassing, but there was nothing I could do about it. I didn't really talk about how I felt with anyone, but I knew that Mum didn't see it as a problem and thought I was too young to start shaving anyway. Besides, it would be embarrassing to ask anyone to help me shave, so I just put up with it.

When I was about fifteen, my sister Collette suggested that I start to get my legs waxed. I have to confess that I was a bit of a wimp and I didn't really like the idea. But I was desperate to feel more confident about myself and agreed to give it a try. Mum didn't see the point but Collette insisted that now I was getting older, I needed to be able to look after my own grooming as much as possible. She booked me an appointment with a beautician she knew and off we went for my first appointment. I was nervous and apprehensive but also looking forward to feeling better about myself. But oh God, did it bloody hurt! Every yank of the strip made me wince in pain and I wondered how much more I could take. It seemed to take forever, but once it was over, I knew it was worth it. I felt so much better without my furry legs and I was really grateful to Collette for suggesting waxing. To this day, I regularly get waxing done and although it has cost me a small fortune over the years, it is well worth it. I don't have the embarrassment of asking anyone to shave me and I get it done when I want to.

I'm in a similar predicament with make-up. It's something that lots of women take for granted and even at school, lots of girls broke the rules to wear it. There was no fear of me ever breaking any rules as it's virtually impossible for me to put it on myself, as much as I would like to. The first time that I remember wearing make-up was my 18th birthday party, when my sisters put it on for me. That in itself is difficult as I have to try really hard to keep my head as still as possible. Believe me, the more I try to keep it still, the more it seems to shake! It's so frustrating at times. Nonetheless, my sisters managed to make me look half decent and I felt really special wearing make-up. From then on, I got some help to put it on for special occasions.

It's easy and quite understandable to take everyday things for granted. But having a disability has meant that I can't take these things as a given and it can be frustrating. I can't always wear make-up if I'm going out, because there might not be anyone around to help me. And I have to plan ahead if I want to get waxing done for an occasion. But despite the mild frustrations,

I wouldn't change my situation. After all, it's quite nice to be pampered and looked after, even if it does hurt like hell!

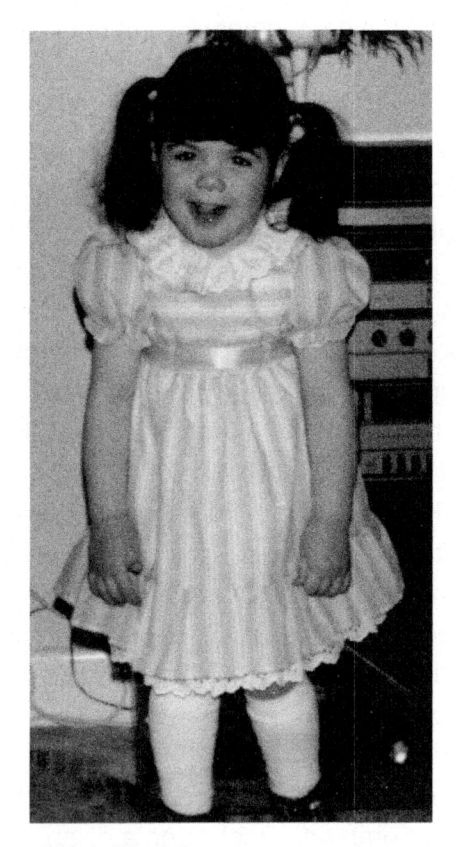

Mum's little doll

Chapter 23
"Bit wobbly on my feet"

I'd been settled in Reading for almost two years and while I'd had my ups and downs at work, my job was going quite well. I was managing a small team, I always had good appraisals and was still really enjoying the job. I had some good friends and regularly went out drinking after work with my best buddy. Life was good, but I began thinking that there was something missing in my life. Love. Dean had been my one serious boyfriend and I missed having someone special in my life. Earlier in the year, I'd gone to Lourdes and although it may sound daft, I'd prayed that I'd meet someone to share my life with, someone that would accept me despite my disability.

Shortly after returning home from that trip, I decided to try online dating again. I say again, because I'd tried it before during my final year at university. But I never really took it seriously – it was just good to have people to chat to. I was always conscious of the fact I didn't really know the people I was talking to – the internet can be devious, or rather the people using it can be! I chatted to a couple of people, but when it came to it, I just didn't trust them to take it any further than online chatting.

I was still sceptical, but I reasoned that if nothing else, I'd be talking to new people and might make some new friends. I really wasn't expecting much, so I only paid for one month's subscription. I sat with my laptop and tried to come up with a profile that wouldn't scare people away! I decided I'd be totally honest, so my profile mentioned my four wheels – if men didn't like that, then I didn't like them! I didn't go into too much detail as I wanted people to focus on me as a person, not my disability.

With my profile and an accompanying photo posted, I began browsing some profiles and occasionally sending winks to a few guys that caught my eye. The website allowed you to view people who had looked at your profile, so I looked at their profiles too. One day shortly after I'd registered, I spotted a guy who called himself 'Thrawg'. He had looked at my profile, but decided not to make contact. How could he resist...

I made a point of never emailing a guy first – if he was keen, he could say hello first. So instead I sent Thrawg a wink, fully expecting it to be ignored. After all, he'd overlooked me once, hadn't he? But he surprised me by sending me an email to introduce himself. I instantly took a shine to him, but wasn't really expecting anything to come from it. I still wasn't sure if I'd be brave enough to actually meet anyone, but I was happy to have someone to chat to and Thrawg seemed genuinely interested in me.

Over the next few days, we emailed each other back and forth, getting to know each other's likes and dislikes. One night, he emailed me asking what my favourite film was. I'm not a film buff and I just went blank. Of all the films I could have said, I replied with *Pretty Woman*, a twenty-year-old romantic comedy! I thought that would be the last I heard from Thrawg: instead he replied, taking the mickey out of me!

As time went by, I felt more comfortable with him and after a few weeks, he said he wanted to meet me. So it was time to tackle something we'd avoided talking about – my CP. As I said, I had mentioned my wheelchair in my profile, but I hadn't gone into any great detail about the CP. So I composed an email explaining my condition and how it affected me. I was brief, but in my opinion, honest and signed off by saying I'd understand if he wanted to leave it there. I really had very little confidence and absolutely no belief that any man would be willing to look beyond my disability.

As I clicked 'send', I really didn't expect a reply. I sat nervously watching my inbox and within minutes I had another email – Thrawg was not a bit concerned about my CP and still wanted to meet me! I was so shocked and surprised, I was convinced I was talking to a con man, or maybe one of my friends was winding me up! But a part of me was over the moon and shortly afterwards, Thrawg told me his real name – Dean. Yet another Dean in my life!

Dean and I had been emailing and texting constantly for at least three weeks. The minute I got back from work, I checked my emails and my phone was practically glued to my hand for most of the day. We'd decided we wanted to meet up the following Saturday, 23rd August. We'd planned where to meet and what we would do. But we still hadn't actually spoken. We were getting on so well and I was terrified that Dean wouldn't be able to understand my speech. What if it put him off and he cancelled our date? What if he made an excuse as to why he couldn't talk to me? All these things played on my mind, but I felt we had to at least speak before we actually met in person.

So I plucked up some courage, took a deep breath and dialled his number. It rang. And again. I waited, wondering if he would answer. I'd told him about my speech and I wondered whether he was as apprehensive as I was. It seemed like ages before he answered. And then what did I do? I bottled it: as soon as he said hello, I hung up! The poor guy, I thought! But I was just so nervous and that makes my speech even worse! I desperately wanted things to go well. Funny way of showing it, eh?

So I took another deep breath and phoned him again. This time I said hello and immediately apologised for hanging up. Dean understood – it had taken me weeks to actually phone him, so he knew what a big deal it was for me. We slowly got chatting and much to my relief, he understood most of what I was saying. We both joked about the other being stood up on Saturday and although instinct told me that he was genuine, I still feared that this was a big joke and that he wouldn't actually turn up.

But I had nothing to fear – from then on we spoke for hours on the phone, racking up £300 phone bills for two months on the trot! Of course, they were his phone bills, but I still felt rather guilty as it wasn't until late September that we were seeing each other most days.

I was a bag of nerves as I set about getting ready to meet for the first time. I had my hair done in town and then my friend came over to help me get ready. I still had my doubts about whether he would actually turn up, but I put my nerves aside and let my excitement take over. I'd brought a new outfit especially – the date had cost me a fortune, so he had better be there!

While getting ready, I'd decided to have a small glass of wine to try and settle my nerves. OK, so make that a large glass and make that two! Alcohol has always calmed me down because, as with everyone, it makes me less self-conscious! It was eventually time to make my way to our meeting place, but I was determined that I wasn't going to be first to arrive. Before I turned the corner and went into the bar, I parked the wheelchair out of view and took a few deep breaths. A tiny part of me wanted to turn around and go home. I thought Dean was too good to be true, but I also knew I had to give him a chance.

One more deep breath, quick brush of my hair and I headed around the corner and into the bar. I was a few minutes late, but I recognised him straight away. I made my way towards him and my fears were laid to rest. He'd turned up and he was a dream come true. The first few minutes were a little awkward as all first dates tend to be, but it wasn't long before we were chatting, laughing and flirting!

Dean was the perfect gentleman and insisted on paying for everything. When our food arrived, he instinctively offered to help me cut it up and again, there was no awkwardness between us. I just knew he was genuine and he understood everything I said. We certainly had a lot to talk about and by the time we said goodnight, we had both committed to seeing each other again.

Four years on and now married, Dean often teases me that before meeting him, I totally misled him. When

I emailed him about my disability, I thought I was being honest and fair by saying: *'I'm a bit wobbly on my feet and my speech can be difficult to understand when I'm stressed...!'*

He jokes with me that this was a total and deliberate distortion of reality! He understands that to me, it's the truth – I don't view my disability as a big issue. However, I do appreciate that to someone who has never encountered CP, that statement does seem slightly misleading!

It was a few weeks and a few dates later when I finally felt comfortable enough to invite Dean to my home. I promised to cook for him on the proviso that he helped me to peel the potatoes, a job I loathed because it was so difficult for me to do. As I prepared the meal, we danced around each other, occasionally making contact as we passed things back and forth. This was the first time we'd been alone together and surprisingly, I felt really comfortable in his company. He didn't seem to notice my clumsy, unladylike movements and I was grateful for his offers of help whenever he noticed me struggling with something.

After our meal, as we cuddled up to watch a film, we had the inevitable, 'where is this relationship going?' conversation. When I'd first met Dean, I hadn't dared to hope that he would be Mr. Right. But now, just a few weeks on, it seemed obvious to us both that we wanted the same thing - a long-term relationship. But I had some concerns. All of my previous relationships had been with guys who also had a disability and it had felt like a level playing field. My strengths had been their weaknesses and vice versa. We had understood each other's physical limitations and there were no unanswered questions hanging between us, or anybody else. But now I worried about how Dean's family and friends would react to the news that his new girlfriend had cerebral palsy and used a wheelchair. He had already told me that his best mate had effectively told him to run a mile. I was hugely insecure and not knowing Dean very well, I thought he might be influenced by their opinions.

'Your friends might think that you'll just turn into my carer and I couldn't blame them,' I said, searching Dean's face for signs of concern. But he really didn't care, as he held me a bit tighter. 'It doesn't matter what they say, it won't change how I feel about you.' Although I felt hugely reassured, I still worried. This was new territory for me and I felt like I'd have to prove myself to his friends and family, prove that I was good enough for him. Prove that I wasn't just looking for a carer, but for a loving relationship, just like anyone else.

It was of course inevitable that Dean would do things to help me, what partner wouldn't want to help? But initially, I felt like I had to prove that I wouldn't be a burden on him.

Chapter 24

A bag of nerves

Dean and I had been inseparable for the past few months and though we had said we'd each have an evening to do our own thing, it never seemed to work out. I knew things were serious – we'd already talked about the future and it was clear that we were committed to each other. And so the inevitable discussion came up – meeting each other's parents. We'd talk about it, but Dean wasn't that bothered either way. I knew he wasn't ashamed of me, but family occasions had never been a priority for him.

He was at the gym one evening, but hadn't let me know when he'd be back and to be honest, I was a little stroppy with him as he hadn't been answering the phone. When we finally spoke, he sensed that he was in the dog house. He had to think quickly and to avoid our first row, he suddenly announced that he was taking me away that weekend – and I'd be meeting his parents. I knew he'd never brought a girl home before so I knew how much it meant. On arriving home, he presented me with the first bunch of flowers he ever bought me and though I was pleased, I said to Dean,

'They're lovely but they are also plastic!' Dean had been oblivious to this and so we laughed for ages! Our first row had been avoided and my irritation with him was soon forgotten! If only plastic flowers could help us avert every row!

I was delighted, to be meeting his parents, excited even but also nervous. What would they make of me? Every parent wants the absolute ideal scenario for their children and in most cases, nobody is ever good enough for them. I understood this and it worried me that Ann and Harry may be resentful, even wary of me and perhaps want different for their son. I voiced my worries to Dean, but he said it didn't matter what anybody thought about our relationship – all that mattered was how he felt about me and his feelings wouldn't be influenced by anyone else. I was reassured, but still nervous.

The weekend arrived and we decided to check into a hotel, rather than stay with Dean's parents. As it was our first meeting, Dean thought we'd all be more comfortable that way. We'd agreed to go and see them on the Saturday and I was a nervous wreck. It seemed to take ages to get from the hotel to their home in Kingsbridge, Devon. Dean had borrowed a satnav from one of his work colleagues and not having used one before, we didn't realise there were different settings. Being set to 'shortest route', it sent us across Dartmoor and down some of the narrowest roads, or should I say dirt tracks, I had ever seen. The so-called shortest route took us an age!

We finally arrived and Dean took me into their house. He briefly introduced us and then went back to the car. I was meeting his parents for the first time, I was super nervous and he'd just sat me down and then left me! Thanks babe, I thought! He'd gone to get the gifts I'd brought for Ann and Harry, but still, he could have waited a while! But Ann and Harry were lovely and I immediately felt welcome in their home. My fears about how they might perceive me were unfounded.

As Dean and I became more comfortable with each other, it was time for me to meet his best friend, Dan. As I said, I knew that Dan had had reservations about me but Dean was adamant that it didn't matter. He was committed to our relationships and nothing anyone else said would change that.

Even so, I was a bag of nerves as Dan arrived at my flat for dinner. It would obviously really help things if we did get on. Just as with Ann and Harry, I needn't have worried. Dan was warm and friendly, though I think at times he struggled with my speech and on occasions, Dean had to translate! The evening went really well and it was a good sign for our relationship, that Dean felt comfortable enough to introduce us.

Shortly afterwards, things were beginning to change at work. We rented office space from the local council and the department that we shared with were undergoing a restructure. We were concerned that the new manager might come in and turf us out. I made it my mission to get this guy on side. As it happened, it wasn't difficult. Barry and I hit it off almost immediately and as soon as I realised that he wasn't giving us our marching orders, we became friends.

His office was next store to ours and I'd often nip next door for a natter. I think my manager soon realised how well we got on and if there was anything we needed from Barry or negotiations to be done, I'd go and sort it out. Barry and I worked well together and found several joint projects, which helped to keep us afloat when our funding began to dry up.

Eventually, Dean and I began socialising with Barry and his partner, Graeme. Luckily, Dean and Graeme got on as well as Barry and I did, and the four of us spend and still do, many happy evenings eating and drinking and putting the world to rights.

While my relationship with Dean flourished, things at work became very stressful. Within months, I'd gone from being committed, happy and motivated to a complete stress-head who no longer cared about anything other than getting the work done and going home.

My manager was a contractor and only worked three days a week. She was very laid back and the two of us worked very well together. She had a very *laissez faire* management style and this worked well for me – I was very driven and we seemed to share the same vision for the organisation, so she let me get on with things. My commitment was obvious, so she didn't have to keep tabs on me.

However, things began to change as the organisation expanded and we took on more staff. I employed a PA through Access to Work - a government scheme which provides support to enable working disabled people to do the bits of their jobs which may otherwise be too difficult. I settled into my new management role well and although there were some initial teething problems, my PA was a big help and I supervised her closely.

I also took over line management of another staff member. I was keen to take on extra responsibility and I thought this was my opportunity to develop my management skills. My manager was supportive of my idea, as were the Board of Trustees. Things went quite well initially, but a few weeks later it became clear there was an issue which needed management intervention. I made a decision which helped the staff member in the short term and gave me time to think about a longer-term solution.

Unfortunately, the Board disagreed with my management approach and decided to intervene. I was disappointed as I knew I could manage the situation and I felt undermined and undervalued when my decision was overruled. I hadn't been allowed to handle the situation myself, despite having proved that I was an effective manager. From then on, my motivation began to dwindle. As much as I loved working with and supporting clients, I became increasingly unhappy.

Fast forward 12 months and the charity was in trouble. The Local Authority had cut our funding, my fixed term contact had ended and I was being employed on a month by month basis, never knowing if my job was safe. This went on for almost six months and it was very stressful and unsettling. Despite the fact that other members of staff had left having found more secure employment, I stayed put and even secured some short term funding which would give us more time to secure the charity's future. Even my manager had decided to leave so I was effectively running the organisation by myself. I know now that my loyalty and commitment were misplaced. In hindsight, I should have taken the opportunity to spread my wings and expand my experience somewhere else, but the job market made that easier said than done and besides, I still believed that new funding would bring me a promotion and an opportunity to progress.

Eventually, after months of uncertainty and never knowing if I would have a job at the end of the month, the charity secured significant funding for a further three years. Thinking this meant my job was finally safe, I was delighted. But my joy was short-lived as, a few days later, I was informed that my job description had been changed and therefore, the role was being treated as a brand new role. In accordance with the funding requirements, the job would be advertised and if I wanted it, I would have to apply for it.

After all those months of expectation, you can imagine my utter frustration and disappointment. This was multiplied when I compared my job description to the 'new' one - the differences were barely noticeable. I was of course allowed to apply for the role, but given my previous managerial conflicts, I wasn't holding out much hope of securing the job - particularly as I was told that there was another, less senior, role that had my name on it.

I felt utterly deflated and I was still the only full-time member of staff keeping the charity going while the new funding was arranged. Stressed and extremely distressed, I ended up crying my eyes out in my GP's office and all I felt was utter despair. I'd worked so hard for the charity, it had been my life and I'd got such satisfaction from helping others. I'd put up with a long period of uncertainty about my job, never once complaining, despite not knowing from one month to the next if I'd be able to pay my bills or feed myself. I'd stayed loyal and yet now it seemed my job was gone anyway. I felt like I couldn't carry on and so the doctor signed me off with stress for two weeks. It was a horrible time in my life - I couldn't eat or sleep and the passion I'd once had for my work had disappeared.

Although I secured an interview for the role, unsurprisingly I wasn't appointed and the job was split between two other candidates. As anticipated, I was offered another role, but it didn't offer any progression, quite the opposite and I knew I was capable of much more. With the job market being so difficult, I felt I had no choice but to accept the job until I could secure something else. I was desperately unhappy and I no longer felt valued or appreciated. I still did my very best for the clients, but I stopped going above and beyond for the organisation.

Chapter 25

Cloud nine

Within weeks of meeting, Dean and I had had a general conversation about our hopes and plans for the future. I was a little wary of this as I didn't want to scare him away, but Dean seemed keen to talk about the future. After some cajoling, I admitted to Dean that one day, I'd like to get married and have children. But this is where our recollections of the conversation differ - significantly! I was merely answering Dean's persistent questions about how I saw my/our future. Dean says it was more an ultimatum along the lines of 'propose to me soon or forget it!'. I maintain that I never would have said that, but if that's how he took it, it certainly didn't scare him off!

We'd been together for just ten months when Dean popped the question. It was our weekly date night and we were heading into town for a Chinese. However, Dean said he wanted to do some shopping beforehand and we arranged to meet in town afterwards. He's pretty useless at keeping secrets, so I had a good idea about the type of shopping he had planned, but I played along! When I met him in town, he was carrying a Sainsbury's bag - not the sort of shopping I'd envisaged, but I didn't say anything. Instead, we made our way to the restaurant and I tried not to get my hopes up. After all, I could've got it all wrong and then I'd end up disappointed.

Throughout the meal, Dean was in a funny mood and kept rummaging in the bag. Every time he reached into it, my heart fluttered just a little bit, but then I'd hide my disappointment as he pulled out leaflets from the bag. As we finished our meal and settled the bill, I began to accept that I'd been wrong - Dean wasn't going to propose. Not tonight anyway.

We arrived home and Dean busied himself in the kitchen while I put my wheelchair on charge and got ready for bed. Then Dean reappeared, with a bulge under his shirt. Having already put the idea of a proposal out of my head, I asked what it was. Then he took a box out from under his shirt and said quite coolly that if I wanted it, I'd have to marry him! Hardly the romantic proposal I'd dreamt of, but I was overwhelmed. Before accepting, I made Dean ask me properly and I squealed with delight as he took the solitaire from the box and put it on my finger.

After being so disappointed that he hadn't proposed over dinner, I was now on cloud nine. But it was typical of Dean - he's not at all traditional and by waiting until we got home, he knew he'd thrown me off the scent. I was absolutely delighted and I couldn't wait to show off my sparkler to anyone who would look! I phoned Ann and Harry to tell them that I would soon be their daughter-in-law and we were seeing my parents that weekend, so I decided I wanted to tell them in person. Mum and Dad were understandably a bit concerned by our speedy engagement, but Dean and I had clicked from day one and although it sounds clichéd, I knew that we were meant to be together and that Dean loved me for who I was despite my disability. That was all I'd ever wished for and I could hardly believe that my dreams were coming true. I was actually getting married and I was over the moon!

We were going to my cousin's wedding two days later and so it was the perfect opportunity to announce our engagement to the family. As we hadn't been together all that long, I knew that my parents would have some concerns, so we reassured them that we were in no rush to set a date. Everyone was happy for us and although we didn't have a date for the wedding, we started saving as much as we could. The wedding that I had in mind wouldn't come cheap!

If ever I needed proof that Dean was with me for better or worse, in sickness and in health, I got it a few months later.

It was the May Bank Holiday weekend and Dean and I were stupidly going food shopping. (These were the days before we discovered online shopping and delivery!) I had just put on my shoes and I decided to go and check what we had in the kitchen, but before I could get that far, I tripped over the foot plates on my wheelchair which was parked in the lounge and ended up in a heap on the floor. In an effort to save myself, I had put my hands out in front of me, but unfortunately, in doing so, I banged my right hand sharply against the metal foot plate. For a moment, I was stunned into silence, but then I screamed in pain as my hand began to throb. One minute I'd been getting ready to go out and the next, I was in agony.

All my life, falling over has been par for the course and I had very rarely done myself real injury. I'd just pick myself up and carry on, quite often even forgetting that I'd fallen. It was amazing that I'd never done myself serious injury and it didn't even occur to me that this time would be any different. Although my hand was still sore, Dean and I proceeded with our plans to go shopping.

As Dean pushed our trolley around the aisles, I used the store's motorised scooter to get around. But as I pushed the controls to operate it, my hand really hurt. I presumed that I had just bruised it and that within a couple of hours, it would be fine again. It was only the next morning, when my hand was twice its usual size and turning purple, that I realised something was wrong.

Dean took one look at my hand and immediately suggested that we go to A&E. I still thought it was just bad bruising, but as I was still in pain, I agreed to go and get it checked out. After all, the hospital was only across the road from where we lived. I hate hospitals and I particularly hate waiting around in them. It was a Bank Holiday so I braced myself for a long wait. However, I was pleasantly surprised that we only waited a couple of hours to be seen. After having my hand examined, I was sent for x-ray, which unfortunately revealed that far from just bruising it, I had in fact broken my hand: I would be in plaster for four weeks. Being my right hand, I was now absolutely 'up the creek without a paddle'.

As I waited to be plastered up, the enormity of what I'd done began to dawn. I wouldn't be able to work in this state as I couldn't even drive my wheelchair or use a computer. As soon as I got my plaster and Dean took me home, I realised just how restricted I was going to be. Simple things that we all take for granted like getting dressed - pulling up jeans and doing up buttons - were now extremely challenging. I couldn't cook meals or make drinks. I couldn't even wash my own hair. All of these things are difficult enough when you have CP, but they were now pretty much impossible.

Dean had just started a new contract in London and

was out for over twelve hours a day - he couldn't be at home to look after me. Before he went to work each day, he'd prepare my breakfast and lunch, as well as enough cold drinks to keep me going all day. When he came home each night, he'd have to cook dinner and then wash up afterwards. There was very little that I could do for myself and for those few weeks, I was totally dependent upon Dean and I felt very guilty, even though I knew it was beyond my control. Travelling to London and back every day was tiring enough, but he also had to do everything in the house. Normally quite independent, I got quite frustrated at not being able to do much for myself.

After many boring days watching daytime TV, my hand slowly healed and although I was still in the cast, I returned to work. Despite everything, I still took my job seriously and hated being off sick for too long. Although I couldn't type much, I had a backlog of clients to see and appointments would keep me busy until my hand healed properly.

Chapter 26
A friendship lost

Just as I had struggled to find a partner, I had always found making true friends quite difficult. Sometimes I felt like a burden and sometimes I felt like people were forcing themselves to make an effort because they felt like they should. Other times, I found it incredibly difficult to reach out to people because I was worried that they wouldn't understand my speech or worst still, people would pretend to understand me and then conversation was too awkward for me to bother with. Though I did have some close friends, it wasn't always easy for me to strike up friendships and there were times when I felt really lonely.

University life had been particularly difficult and I'd often been quite lonely. I was delighted when I secured my work placement and I saw moving to Reading as a fresh start and an opportunity to perhaps make some friends. The office where I was based was friendly and I soon found myself immersed in the office banter. There were quite a few people of my age and I soon got to know them, particularly a girl called Lucy.

Lucy was a few years older than me and had worked in our office for a while before I arrived. She was welcoming and funny and I warmed to her almost immediately. She seemed happy to take me under her wing, telling me what was what and we'd have a natter in the staff kitchen at lunchtime. Eventually we started going out for drinks after work and nattering about men and family, as well drinking our way into the night. Lucy listened as I confided my fears of never finding a man who would accept my situation and I sympathised when she told me about her latest row with her boyfriend. We became really close and Lucy became the one person I'd turn to if I had a problem and vice versa. We were as thick as thieves and in the summer of 2007, we booked a holiday to Corfu. It was my first holiday without the family and I was so pleased that Lucy wanted to go with me, despite the fact she would have to push me around in my wheelchair. It just didn't bother her and I knew we were firm friends, it felt good to finally have found a friend who I could talk to and have a laugh with.

We had an amazing holiday, relaxing in the sun and having a laugh. I can't remember why but we brought a Sponge Bob Square Pants helium balloon (probably when we were in a drunken stupor!) and tied it to my wheelchair. From then on, there were three of us on that holiday and it was a talking point everywhere we went. We only parted with Sponge Bob when we were about to board the plane to come home!

As I said, life was good but Lucy knew that I was lonely. I'd told her about my ex, Dean and though I knew now that he really wasn't right for me, I longed to meet someone new who would be accepting of my condition and who would love me just for who I was. We'd been on nights out, in the hope that I might meet someone special but I knew deep down that I wouldn't meet Mr. Right in some loud, busy nightclub. My speech was hard to understand at the best of times and it was even harder for me to make myself understood in that kind of environment. So when I started online dating, Lucy was as supportive as ever. She was the first person I told when I met 'Thrawg' and she shared my excitement as we exchanged emails and texts, and eventually arranged our first date, which Lucy agreed to help me get ready for.

My relationship with Dean blossomed and, as any best friend would be, Lucy seemed happy for me. Despite the fact that I was now in a committed and happy relationship, I was determined to maintain my independence and still saw Lucy as much as I did before. I wasn't the type of girl to ditch her friends in favour of a man. As Dean and I moved in together, Lucy and her boyfriend finally split up and we helped her move into a new pad. I was there as much as I could be to help her over the split and despite her pain, she was happy for me when Dean proposed.

But then, out of nowhere, everything suddenly went wrong. I was at Lucy's one Saturday evening and we were having our usual weekly natter over a few drinks. Slightly tipsy, we started talking about the wedding, at which she was to be my bridesmaid, and I explained how I'd started doing some walking in the park to try and strengthen my legs. I desperately wanted to be able to walk down the aisle and realising how much it meant to me, Dean had offered to help me with my walking. Every day, I was able to walk just a little bit further and I was so proud of what I was achieving. But Lucy didn't seem so pleased.

'He's pushing you to do things you're not capable of. Stop putting him on a pedestal,' she suddenly ranted, making very little sense. She continued saying that it was Dean pushing me to exercise and that I was blind to how he was trying to control and change me. Her strange outburst shocked me and I explained that it was my idea, but Lucy wouldn't accept it. We had never argued about anything before and I was desperately trying to defuse the situation, believing that our friendship would eventually win out. But there was no talking to Lucy and as tears trickled down my face, she phoned Dean and asked him to collect me. It was like Lucy had completely changed in the space of minutes and nothing I said made any difference. She refused to accept that I was capable of making my own decisions and that I'd never allow Dean, or indeed any man, to control me.

So in a blink of an eye, after six years, our friendship was over. I thought that maybe when Lucy sobered up, she might realise how wrong she'd been, but she refused to speak to me and I was devastated. I'd lost my best friend over a stupid, drunken row and for months I felt like I'd been bereaved. My best friend was gone and for the life of me, I didn't understand why: I kept wishing I could turn the clock back and replay that evening differently.

To this day, I don't really understand how we could be as close as sisters and then fall out so spectacularly over nothing. At the time, our lives were going in different directions; I was about to get married while Lucy had recently ended a long-term relationship. It was a period of change for us both and I often wonder whether this contributed to how Lucy was feeling. Perhaps she felt we would drift apart anyway. I often think about her and the friendship that we shared. I laugh at some of our memories and I sometimes shed a tear for the loss of a friendship that I cherished. I might never know the reasons, but I hope she's found as much happiness as I have.

Chapter 27
An Irish tradition

Although I'd always dreamt about getting married, I never really thought it would happen. Now that it was, I had my heart set on the fairy-tale wedding.

After lots of discussion, both with each other and my parents, we decided on an Irish Wedding, back in Sligo. There were a couple of reasons for this, the main one being that you just can't beat an Irish Wedding! They typically go on for at least two days and are the best craic ever! We'd already decided on a September wedding and had a short-list of hotels. We trawled through many brochures, menus and websites before finally booking the Clarion in Sligo.

Dean and I made a couple of trips over to Sligo to confirm the venue and meet with the photographer, and I made a couple of trips on my own so that I could go shopping for 'The Dress' with my Mum and sisters. As I said, I was absolutely determined to be just like any other bride and actually *walk* down the aisle. As I'd tried to explain to Lucy, Dean and I had started going to our local park so that I could practise walking and build up the strength in my legs. I spend so much time in my wheelchair that my muscles are quite weak. At first, I could barely walk ten yards without getting tired and out of breath. I also leaned heavily on Dean for support. I began to wonder if my dream of *walking* down the aisle was just that. A dream.

But Dean provided lots of support and encouragement and we went to the park most days after work. Within just a few weeks, I could do a whole lap of the park without stopping. I still got out of my breath but my legs were definitely getting stronger. I was so proud of myself as I realised that my dream of walking down the aisle could definitely become a reality, but I was still scared that I'd end up falling over. I needed my dress to be practical, as well as stunning. I tried on dozens of dresses and in the end, I was torn between two. Such an important decision!

After a few months of deliberating back at home, I returned to Ireland to make my final decision - a beautiful ivory, halter-neck dress with lots and lots of lace! Trying it on for the second time, I knew it was the one and that it could easily be taken up to ensure I wouldn't trip.

Now that everything was falling into place, I was like a kid waiting for Christmas! The third of September just couldn't come soon enough and I began counting the days until I became Mrs Blackborough!

But before that, Dean was heading off to Wales for his Stag weekend. Barry and Graeme are some of our best friends and had been appropriately warned – look after my hubby-to-be or else. There were still lots of jobs to be done for the wedding so I knew the weekend would fly by. But there was one special task that I wanted to complete while Dean was away as I wanted it to be a surprise for everyone on our wedding day. I'd been thinking about it for weeks, trying to get it just right in my head. I was agonising over every word, every line, but now I had the opportunity to get it down on paper and practise it aloud. After some hours, I was happy with my efforts.

I would have all my family and friends in one place and it was the perfect occasion to pay tribute to each and every one of them. It was an opportunity to publicly thank my family and friends for their incredible love and support. I'd always felt so blessed and I wanted everyone to know how important they were to me and of course, I wanted to do something a bit different and memorable for Dean. He'd made my life complete and I wanted to shout it from the rooftops.

Finally, Saturday 3 September dawned and I could hardly believe it. I was getting married. TODAY!!! Excitement and anticipation filled our family home in Sligo and, just like an excited kid waiting for Santa, I couldn't wait for the day to begin. I nestled under the duvet until I couldn't bear it any longer and then I jumped out of bed as if it were on fire. I danced into my en suite and started the water running for my shower. As the warm water washed over me, I wondered if the day ahead would go as we'd planned. By the end of that day, I'd be a married woman. A new chapter was starting in my life and I couldn't wait to turn the page.

The morning passed in a blur of activity and excitement as I counted down the minutes until I would become Mrs Blackborough. When I arrived for my hair appointment, the small salon was already full of wedding guests, many of whom were new to Sligo and had accepted Mum's recommendation for a hairdresser. Above the hum of hairdryers, chatter and laughter filled the small salon and it felt like the celebrations had already begun. I could hardly stop grinning as my hair was styled and my tiara was pinned firmly in place - I felt like a princess already! I chatted away to the stylist and said hello and goodbye as my wedding guests arrived and then left the salon.

My hair complete, it was left to my brother James to collect me and take me back to the house. Quite appropriately, the car radio blared with the latest Bruno Mars tune, *'Marry You'*. I'd not heard it before, but on the short journey home, we sang along and I couldn't stop smiling! I was on an absolute high and as we arrived home, the excitement escalated as my bridesmaids and flower girls arrived and we all started getting ready. My sister had arranged for her best friend to do my make-up and the photographer arrived to capture me getting ready as we sipped Bucks Fizz. She'd already seen my husband-to-be and assured me that following his boys' night out he was in one piece and all ready for the ceremony. Phew! Like most brides, I'd been fretting about what the lads might get up to, but I'm told that the boys' antics that night will forever remain a secret!

Aside from the necessary hairdo, on this *very* special occasion my sister Martina had made another fashion suggestion. From a young age, I'd always worn glasses. At first it was just for school, looking at the blackboard and watching television, but as time went on, I wore them all the time. I didn't particularly mind, but it was a pain having to clean them, especially as I can be quite heavy handed! I've broken my glasses on several occasions. So with the wedding approaching, Martina suggested that I wear contact lenses for the big day. She knew it would make me feel better if I didn't have to be concerned with cleaning my glasses. Plus, given the Irish weather, I'd be better off wearing contacts in case it rained. At first, I thought she was mad: how would I be able to put contact lenses in? But Martina said she would be happy to put them in for me. I was still unsure, as I didn't like the idea of anything in my eyes, but I agreed to go to the opticians for a contact lens assessment.

The optician was happy for my sister to help me, but she would have to be shown how to do it, so a few days before the wedding we went into the optician in Sligo. It took a few attempts to get them in, but eventually, we got there. It felt really weird being able to see without having to wear my glasses, but it was brilliant! I looked and felt so much better without my glasses and lots of people complimented me. But because I couldn't put them in myself, I'd never even considered lenses until now. I was so grateful to Martina for suggesting it and offering to help me. It made me feel so much more confident on such a special day.

With my make-up done, all that was left to do was to step into my dress. I felt absolutely amazing and at times, I wondered if I was just dreaming. But no, thankfully this was real and I was so excited. I thought I'd feel a bit nervous but all I felt was pure elation. After clock-watching all morning, it was finally time to make the short journey with Dad to the church.

The church was packed and some guests were standing at the back, waiting for me to make my entrance. I said a silent prayer to help me make it down the aisle and the Wedding March began. My bridesmaids and flower girls began walking down the aisle in front of me and I held Dad's arm tightly as I began walking towards the altar. Each step I took was slow and careful but I couldn't stop beaming as my friends and family turned to watch. As we approached the altar, Dean peered down the aisle, and as Dad gave me away, he whispered, 'He's here Aideen, Dean's here.' It was a wonderful moment.

As Dad gave my hand to Dean and shook his hand, I took Dean's hand in mine and glanced around at my family and friends. In that moment, I had absolutely no doubt that I was the luckiest girl alive. I had the most supportive and loving family I could ask for, the most amazing friends and, in less than an hour, I'd have a wonderful husband to add to my blessings. At that moment, life really couldn't have been any better.

As Dean isn't religious, I'd spent hours carefully planning the wedding ceremony and after picking out some of my favourite readings and hymns, I'd asked some of our closest friends and family to do the readings and prayers. Then came the important bit - making our vows. I was so happy and emotional, I was worried that I might not be able to get the words out, but I managed to keep my tears at bay as I promised to love and cherish Dean for the rest of my life. A roar of applause went up as we were pronounced man and wife.

I was on an absolute high. I was now a married woman and the happiest that I'd ever been. The wedding had gone without a hitch, we'd got some wonderful photos and now we were sitting down to the wedding breakfast.

But before the food, we'd agreed to do the speeches – mainly so that Dad could enjoy his meal without being full of nerves about his speech.

Dan, Dean's best man, had run his speech by me a few days earlier, so I knew his would be short and sweet. Just as well. At my sister's wedding nine years earlier, my dear Dad had given a lovely speech which lasted over half an hour and now the stopwatches were at the ready! Though he was nervous, Dad did us all proud with a heart-warming and at times funny speech. Though he acknowledged that life had not always been easy for me, his pride in me was clear. The speech was very emotional and as the tears gathered in my eyes, I feared I wouldn't be able to deliver my own surprise!

Dad topped twenty-five minutes and although I knew everyone was hungry, I think they were able to forgive him. Next up was the groom. Now Dean is not a naturally social person so I must admit to being worried about his speech. But I needn't have worried. Just like my Dad, my new husband did me so proud. We had written a list of about a thousand Thank-Yous and I was terrified that we'd forget someone. By the time Dean had finished, I thought I might get lynched if I delayed the meal any longer.

Everyone was surprised as the Master of Ceremony handed me the microphone and a folded piece of paper. I began with a promise: to only take two minutes – unlike the boys! And then I began to read:

Though it's not tradition
for the bride to make a speech
I just have a few words to say,
on this, our wedding day.

I've always been so blessed,
with all that I've been given,
God really has been good
beginning with my childhood.

Today I give heartfelt praise and thanks
to my dear Mum and Dad
who have always been there
with never-ending love and care.

I send my love and admiration
to my sisters and little bro,
no girl could ever ask for more
of the siblings that I adore.

I thank God for so many friends and family,
for the love and laughs we share,
I thank you for being here today
for always being there, come what may.

And now I've been blessed to find a husband
a best friend to see me through,

> you really are my soul mate
> I've known since our first date.
>
> I pray our life is long and happy,
> that our dreams will be fulfilled ,
> Today is the best of my life
> and I thank God I'm your wife.
>
> So now all that remains to say
> is it's time to celebrate,
> fill your glasses and have some fun
> the speeches are finally all done!

As I read, I glanced around at my family, friends and then my husband, but not for too long – I had to keep going before the emotion got to me. Just before the final verse, a roar of applause went up and I was finding it hard to finish. But as I read that last line, I finally looked at the crowd around me and hoped they realised what they all meant to me. I don't care what anyone says – in that moment, I was the happiest and luckiest girl alive.

With the speeches finished, it was time to party! My Mum had decorated the room with balloons, Dean's Dad had made us a brilliant four tier wedding cake and Martina had prepared a spread of cakes and chocolates to give our guests an extra treat. Everything was absolutely perfect and after all the emotional speeches, we kicked off the night with our first dance - Michael Buble's *'Crazy Love'*. Knowing it would be difficult for me to dance in my dress, Dean lifted me into his arms and we swayed across the dance floor until he couldn't hold me up anymore! It was another wonderful moment of a wonderful day. We continued to dance the night away and I made sure to go around every table to thank our guests for coming. That took quite some time! Then the evening was interrupted by some strange guests.

There is a unique and rather eccentric tradition in the West of Ireland and no wedding is complete without it - The Straw Boys. You might well ask who the Straw Boys are, but that would be a very difficult question to answer, as nobody really knows! If you pushed me for an explanation though, I'd have to say this: The Straw Boys are a group of mad hatters who disguise their identities with straw hats (covering their faces) and travel around the West of Ireland gate crashing weddings! They bring with them songs and dance, as well as many best wishes for the bride and groom. They usually have inside information in order to write a 'Pass' for the happy couple and ours went something like this:

> We've marched in from Cloonacool and on through Ballisodare
> To find this happy couple; we've been searching everywhere.

We walked through bogs, bet off cross dogs to find this man and wife. We've come to wish them Both Good Luck and a long and happy life!

We have duties to dispense and blessings to bestow
Anyone could get a mention, you'd just might never know
So clear the floor and lend an ear to what we have to say
We won't say no to Liam's mountain dew or Deirdre's cups of tea.

To Aideen and her unrivalled beauty - this toast I will propose
She could be in Tralee any year as England's finest Rose
Independent and intelligent, a great favourite with the clan
Sure no doubt the buck that gets her will be a lucky man!
And so Dean Blackborough from over the water
Came to court Bill Jack's lovely grand daughter.

Soon there was talk of wedding bells and celebrations
Of cakes and dresses, of fancy cars and invitations!
Collete said she'd do the dinner and dessert would be banoffi
Martina offered chocolate and lots and lots of coffee.
Deirdre said she'd deck the halls and brighten up the room
She had lots of party banners and a special offer on balloons!
And the happy day arrived when the plans all came together
With prayers to the Infant of Prague and Granny for good weather.

Folks flew in from Reading and Devon and even further a-field
All piled together in Calry for the festivities and the feed!
Everyone had such a lovely day; in the memory it will linger;
Aideen has her brand new man and a ring upon her finger

The couple were so happy they said t'was such a thrill
As they feck off back to England and leave Seamus with the bill!

Dean and Aideen; their names they are so alike
Their children might be B deen and C deen and suchlike.
So let the Straw Boys work our spell for we will soon be gone
But get ready for a christening for our magic won't take long!
We wish ye health and wealth and joy
And then of course a baby boy!
And when his hair begins to curl
We wish ye then a baby girl!
And when she is fit to feed the hens
We wish ye then a pair of twins!

May your joys be many and your burdens be few
And may the luck of the Straw Boys be always with you!

from The Cloonacool Straw Boys –
September 3rd 2011

As the boys finished The Pass, I was laughing and crying, as were most of our guests. The Straw Boys were absolutely brilliant and everyone had great fun. We sang and danced with them, as is tradition and I really didn't want the night to end. But we knew the celebrations would continue tomorrow, as Mum and Dad were throwing a party for us at their house. It gave us more time to spend with all our guests, many of whom had travelled a good distance to be with us. It really made me realise what a great family and group of friends we had and I was so thankful.

It still hadn't quite sunk in that I was now Mrs Blackborough and as we headed back to England a few days later, I was still on cloud nine! And we still had our honeymoon to look forward to. We'd booked it even before we'd booked the wedding reception as we knew exactly what we wanted - a twelve night cruise around the Mediterranean. Just like the wedding, it was perfect.

Neither of us had done a cruise before so we weren't sure what to expect. But we weren't disappointed. We spent twelve days cruising the Mediterranean, eating wonderful food and being entertained from morning to night. The cruise was the perfect choice for us as the ship was totally accessible and when Dean was preoccupied with his laptop, (yes even on honeymoon!), I was able to go and be pampered in the spa. It was truly a wonderful holiday and was the perfect end to a magical few weeks.

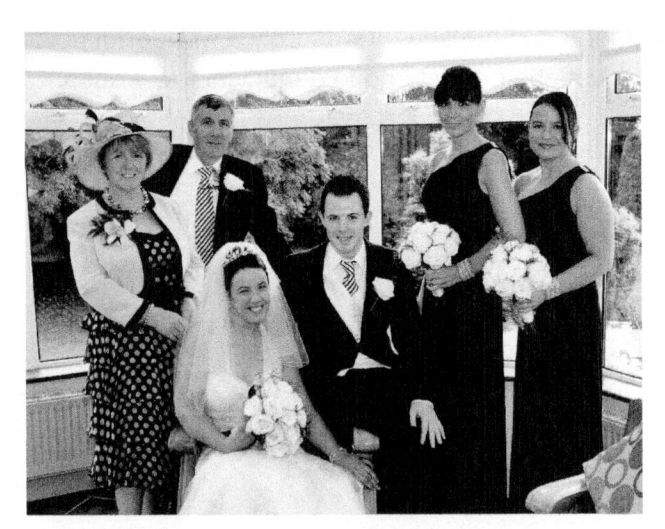

With the family, just before becoming Mrs Blackborough

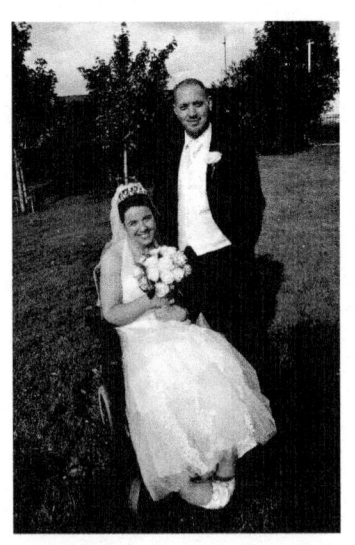

I felt like the happiest girl alive

Chapter 28

Flyinglady

Shortly after the wedding, Dean and I made a major decision. We were going to move up north, back to where I grew up in Great Barr. Next door in fact. A few months before, my Dad had brought our old neighbours' house as a renovation project. He asked us if we'd like to live there and after some serious consideration, we decided to take it.

I was still unhappy at work, nothing had improved and I was stuck in a rut. There were no new opportunities and if truth be told, I didn't feel like I was being valued. I knew if we moved to Birmingham, it was the perfect opportunity for me to develop my own business - Flyinglady Training. I wanted to really focus on what I was good at and what I enjoyed - training people. It was the aspect of my job that I really enjoyed and I knew I was good at it. Flyinglady would focus on Equality and Diversity training and while I worked my notice, I spent my evenings writing and preparing my own courses, as well as getting a website up and running. (Take a look at www.flyinglady-training.co.uk)

Although tinged with sadness, it was a huge relief when I finally finished at work in December 2011, after almost 7 years. I'd spent far too long getting upset and stressed with things that I had no control over and I knew it was time to move on. The house took longer to finish than we had anticipated, but we finally moved in the May and I threw myself into Flyinglady.

It wasn't easy to get established, particularly at a time when most budgets were being cut and staff training fell off the priority lists of almost all organisations. I kept trying everything I could think of: mail shots, cold calling, networking meetings. I tried it all, but progress was slow. It was frustrating and I wasn't sure what I could do. Although I obviously wanted a profitable business, some of my personal experiences as a disabled person made me want to make a difference to benefit other people and so I switched my focus.

As a kid, Great Barr seemed like a great little spot. It was only now, as an adult in a wheelchair, that I realised how inaccessible it really was. Despite the Equality Act 2010, only a handful of the local shops were fully accessible to disabled people and I became increasingly frustrated. With lots of encouragement from Dean, I launched a campaign - 'Making Great Barr *great* for Disabled People.'

I began by visiting all of the shops, all eighty-one of them. I assessed how accessible they were - either fully accessible, not accessible or partly accessible. I also gathered other information including whether or not the retailers displayed accessibility signage or had a doorbell for disabled customers to attract attention. My research concluded that:

- Only 29% of the shops were fully accessible to disabled customers, despite the legal requirements placed upon businesses to make their goods and services accessible;

- Less than 10% of the retailers displayed any kind of accessibility signage;

- Only 2 of the 81 retailers had a doorbell which could be used to attract attention.

Accessibility in Great Barr was extremely poor and I decided to compile a report which would highlight the accessibility issues and make some recommendations for change. Once it was complete, a friend helped me to hand-deliver a copy of the report to each of the eighty-one businesses and I sent a copy to the local council, our local MP, and all the local newspapers. The response we received was extremely mixed. Some retailers welcomed the report and promised to read it. Others weren't very interested at all, saying they'd read it 'if they got time.' One retailer, who shall remain unnamed, didn't seem to want the report and as we were leaving, threw it across the floor! Needless to say that this particular shop is extremely inaccessible and may benefit from reading the report's recommendations!

On the day that I released the report, the local newspaper phoned me and said that they wanted to run a story about the campaign. I can't tell you how excited I was! While I'd been in the newspaper several times before when I'd been employed in Reading, I'd never been in it for something I'd done by myself. The newspaper took a few details and sent a photographer out to take my picture. I'd expected a small article, squeezed in between all the other local stories. When the newspaper came out a few days later, I was even more excited - I was on the front page! I was ecstatic! It was quite a lengthy write up, which included snippets from my report, as well as some quotes which I'd provided.

I was convinced that the newspaper report would help the campaign to gather pace, but I soon began to realise that I had a major battle on my hands. As I said, the report had been delivered to eighty-one retailers, but only one formally responded, by phoning me to explain that the report would be forwarded to their head office. The council's access department didn't respond at all and I had to write to my MP a second time to get a response. It was becoming obvious that accessibility, although a legal requirement, was way down everyone's list of priorities.

It took six months to get a response from the council, but when it came I wasn't filled with confidence. Although they acknowledged that there were problems, they didn't seem overly eager to address them. They requested the specific data about which shops were inaccessible and said that they would remind them of their responsibilities under the Equality Act 2010. But they also tried to say that Building Regulations only required *new builds* to be fully accessible - essentially excusing old buildings from making any effort.

I provided the data which they had requested and hoped that a reminder from the council would push the retailers in the right direction. But then I received a further letter from the council, in which they did a complete U-turn. They said that they didn't have the resources to send out reminders, but that I was free to do so! The cheek! That was effectively what I'd done by compiling the report and look where it had got me...

The council were just not interested in my cause so I wrote to the Minister for Disabled People and when he failed to even respond, I wrote to David Cameron. I knew there was little that he could do about such a local issue, but at this point, I felt like I was banging my head firmly against a brick wall and nobody seemed to be listening. David Cameron at least responded by batting it back to a department I had already contacted, but they *still* haven't done anything.

It's a battle which I'm still fighting.

As well as working on the business and fighting for much needed change, I enjoyed our new home and the extra space that we now had.

Our new kitchen was much bigger than the one we'd had in the flat and I was eager to put it to good use. It was Dean's birthday and as he was at work, I planned to make him a surprise birthday cake. I don't normally attempt such things when I'm on my own, just in case. I'm not sure what got into me, but I must have been feeling especially confident.

I got everything out that I would need and began preparing the cake mix. This can be difficult for me due to my lack of dexterity, but my friend Ian had brought me an electric whisk which made things much easier. I also had a little gadget to help me safely crack the eggs so everything was going wonderfully. The cake mix was ready and as carefully as I could, I scooped it into the cake tin. I was so proud of my achievement; it was rare for me to bake without some kind of incident or without the kitchen looking like a bomb site. I'd done well, even if I do say it myself.

But then, you guessed it, disaster struck! As I

lowered the cake tin into the oven, I knocked the bottom of the tin, which flipped and the cake mixture went EVERYWHERE! All over the oven, kitchen floor and even splashed up the kitchen cupboards. I didn't know whether to laugh or cry, so out of pure frustration, I let out a scream! I'd got so close to making a cake without any assistance and now my efforts had been in vain.

As I set about cleaning up the mess, I began to see the funny side, but I was still disappointed that Dean wouldn't be coming home to the smell of a lovely, homemade cake. Instead, I phoned him to tell him what I'd done and vowed to make another cake over the weekend, when he'd be home to help put it in the oven.

I do enjoy cooking and baking, but as this incident shows, it can be hard work as well as frustrating. I have accumulated gadgets which make life easier such as an electric potato peeler and a chopping board which has the knife attached to it so that I have more control over it. But nonetheless, I've learnt my lesson and only take over the kitchen when there's someone around to assist in an emergency!

Chapter 29

The green light

I'd always wanted to be a mum. When I was young and unconcerned by practicalities, I just assumed that I would live the fairy tale; find the man of my dreams, have several children and live happily ever after. Wasn't that what most little girls dreamt of?

As I grew older, my desire to live this dream never faltered, but with maturity came realism. I wondered whether I would be physically capable of carrying a child, and even if I was, how would I cope looking after a baby? There were things I couldn't even do for myself; how on earth would I meet the needs of a demanding newborn, an adventurous toddler? I kept my thoughts to myself as I was terrified that someone would confirm my fears and say, 'No, don't be silly, you wouldn't be able to cope with a baby'.

But the longing for a child was always there and when my sister, Collette, had her first baby, the desire to be a mummy myself intensified. I remember going home to Sligo to visit Luke, my first nephew. He was just a few days old and as I held him in my arms, treating him like a china doll, I silently hoped and prayed that one day I'd be blessed with a baby of my own. I still couldn't bring myself to voice what was on my mind, for fear that my dream might be crushed.

Then one day, I was chatting with Mum and Collette when the subject of having children came up. Now was my opportunity and I decided to seize it. 'Mum, do you know of any reason why *I* wouldn't be able to have children?' I asked as casually as possible. I was worried about what her response would be, but I had to know and I thought maybe she knew something that I didn't. I'd often thought about the court case, all those years ago and wondered whether my future prospects had been forecast. I knew that evidence had been given stating that it was unlikely that I'd ever be able to drive a car. I wondered whether the prospect of me ever being a parent had been discussed.

'I don't see why you wouldn't be able to, it's not like you're not able to push, is it?' Quietly, I was filled with relief. Mum hadn't ripped my dream to shreds as I'd feared; she'd given me silent hope. Of course, I knew that it wasn't solely about being physically capable of carrying a child and giving birth, as difficult as that would inevitably be. I also worried about the practicalities of looking after a child. Through my work, I met another disabled lady and soon learnt that she had a daughter. Although our disabilities were totally different, she had a similar level of mobility to me. One day, I bumped into her on my day off and as we sat having a coffee, I plucked up the courage and politely asked her how she found being a disabled parent. I was wary as I didn't want to pry or offend her, but her response was very encouraging. She explained how even from a young age, her daughter had adapted to her needs, almost sensing that Mummy needed a little extra help. She'd always found her own way of doing things, however difficult and as children so willingly do, her daughter accepted and adapted to her. Her experiences inspired me.

Dean and I had talked about having children just a few weeks after we met. Dean knew how much I would like to have children and although he wasn't as keen as I was, he wasn't completely averse to the idea. But despite Mum's comments, we both had real concerns about whether I would be physically able to cope with pregnancy and the effect it could have on my condition. We wanted to have all the facts from an expert before we started trying for a baby.

But hours on the internet proved fruitless. A visit to my GP produced just an NHS Direct number. I emailed specialist organisations and got no response. Surely it wasn't this difficult? I was looking for an obstetrician with a particular interest in disabled women.

But my search for information was frustrating; did

women who had CP choose not to get pregnant? I emailed the Disabled Parents Network and got no reply. I tried a hundred different search terms and still got nowhere. Even Dean, who is a whizz on the internet, couldn't find anything of any use. Then I made a decision. If the NHS didn't offer specialist support, then we'd have to go private to get the answers we desperately needed. As soon as my mindset changed, so did the results.

Within a few minutes, I found the Harley Street Centre for Women. After reading their website, I'd found an obstetrician who specialised in complex pregnancies. Surely he'd be able to help? As I dialled the number, I was shaking with both apprehension and excitement. This could be my first step towards fulfilling yet another dream. I briefly explained my situation to the receptionist and asked if Mr O'Brien would be prepared to meet us. The afternoon dragged as the receptionist promised to discuss my case with Mr O'Brien and give me a call back.

When the phone eventually rang, I was thrilled – Mr O'Brien was prepared to see us. You might say of course he was, for a hefty consultation fee. And that was my ultimate fear. What if we saw him and he couldn't help? Worse, what if he said pregnancy wasn't recommended for women like me? He could take his fee and break my heart.

Dean couldn't take a day off until his current contract ended, so I booked the appointment for the middle of March when I knew he'd be free. For the next seven weeks, I was both excited and scared. I knew that if we got bad news, I'd be absolutely devastated. I tried to prepare myself for the worst, just in case. The night before our appointment I hardly slept. I just wanted to know if it was possible that one day I might be a mother. Yes or no. That was all I needed.

Arriving at the clinic, we filled out some forms and then we waited to be called. It seemed like hours before Mr O'Brien opened the door and ushered us in. I immediately liked him and he was Irish, so that put me at ease! Although I was a bag of nerves, I managed to make myself understood as I explained how much we wanted to start a family and were searching for answers about how pregnancy may affect me. I had a million questions which started to spill out but Mr O'Brien put my brakes on. A medical history would kind of help him answer my questions!

As he asked me some questions, I began to relax. My answers weren't concerning him and he was being very positive. Then he gave his verdict: I was as capable of having a baby as any other woman and I wouldn't be at any higher risk. A big surprise came when he said a natural birth shouldn't be ruled out, providing the latter stages of pregnancy didn't leave me too exhausted.

As he spoke, I was grinning from ear to ear and I could have cried. My next dream could actually become reality.

Chapter 30

Two pink lines

It was shortly after our first wedding anniversary. I'd been checking the calendar, counting the days. Double checking. I'd done all this before, several times over the past six months and I'd always ended up disappointed. So I didn't dare to hope this time. Not yet.

I couldn't think about anything else. I wondered and I pondered. Finally, when I couldn't take it anymore, I slipped the box out of my bedside drawer and locked myself in the bathroom. In just two minutes, I would know for sure if my dream had come true. As I took the pregnancy test, I tried not to get my hopes up, but at the same time, I kept whispering, 'Please God, please.'

Two minutes felt like two hours as I waited for the result. Finally, I allowed myself to look down.

Two pink lines. Yes, TWO PINK LINES! I couldn't believe my eyes. I was pregnant.

I could hardly believe it as I sat staring at the test. I'd done several tests over the past few months and each one had left me disappointed. Now, according to this test, my dream had become a reality and I couldn't believe it.

I decided to jump in the shower until I worked out what to do next. As I let the warm water wash over me, I wondered if I was dreaming. But once I got out of the shower, I checked the test again and the two pink lines remained. I decided to not tell Dean until I'd had it confirmed by the doctor, partly because I didn't want to get excited until I had it confirmed.

Dean was working from home at the time so I phoned the doctor under the pretence that I needed my flu jab and unusually, they had a free appointment that afternoon. The hours until my appointment dragged and I was finding it difficult to concentrate on anything other than the fact that I *might* be pregnant. When I finally walked into the doctor's office, I was shaking like a leaf as I explained that I'd done a pregnancy test and it was positive. The doctor informed me that pregnancy tests rarely give a wrong positive result and after a few questions, a smile spread across his face as he said, 'Congratulations, you're five weeks pregnant'. I've never wanted to kiss a doctor as much as I did right then. With tears of joy in my eyes, I made my way out to reception to book an appointment with the midwife.

I was still in shock as I told the receptionist that I was pregnant, but I was shocked further by her response. 'Oh dear,' she said sympathetically, as she wrongly assumed that the pregnancy was a mistake. I was too elated to let her bring me down, but it made me fearful of how other people would respond to my news. I decided not to dwell on that now, as there was only one person I wanted to tell.

Before I could go home and tell Dean, I had to call and see Mary. Her sister had sadly lost her battle with cancer that morning and I wanted to see how she was holding up. It felt wrong being so happy while Mary was so sad and I tried to forget my news as I sympathised with her. I knew that in a few weeks, Mary would be overjoyed by my news, but until then I had to try and keep it to myself.

By the time I arrived home, Dean had finished work for the day and was in the kitchen, preparing dinner. I was trying really hard to act normally, as I'd hoped to tell him the news as we ate dinner, but as soon as he asked me how my appointment had gone, I couldn't wait any longer.

'You're going to be a Daddy!' I blurted out. Dean rarely gets excited about anything, other than technology and as continued chopping vegetables, he didn't even look up as he replied, '*I knew that already.*'

Cool as a cucumber! Amazed at his calmness, I enquired how on earth he knew when I didn't even know until an hour ago. Being a tech nerd, Dean had installed an app on my tablet so I could track my cycle. Over the past few days, the tablet had been glued to my hand as I'd checked the dates over and over again, making sure they were right before I wasted yet another pregnancy test. Although I hadn't said anything to him, I had underestimated how observant my husband was and he'd put two and two together.

As I said, it can be difficult to get Dean to react to anything but I knew deep down, he was as pleased as I was. We agreed to keep the news to ourselves for a few weeks, at least until I'd had the first appointment with my midwife. We needed time to let things sink in before sharing the news with friends and family, some of whom would inevitably have concerns about my being pregnant. I wanted to enjoy the realisation of my dream before dealing with everybody else's reactions.

My first meeting with the midwife was at home a few weeks later. Being an advocate of equality, I should know better than to scupper to stereotypes, but on this occasion, I couldn't help myself. I painted a picture in my head of an old battle-axe who would look down on me and judge me incapable of being a mum. I was convinced I would get disapproving looks, patronising advice and perhaps even worse. While I was extremely excited about my first appointment, I was equally anxious.

As soon as I met Corrine, all my fears were laid to rest. She was a little older than me and had three children of her own. She was friendly and approachable and I knew I'd feel safe and reassured in her hands. During that first appointment, I felt so comfortable that I shared my biggest fear. 'I'm afraid that people will think I'm incapable and will take my baby away,' I confessed, quite tearfully.

Even before I fell pregnant, this was something I'd thought about and now, I struggled to push such thoughts away. I'd read so many stories about parents having their children taken away from them, some for no good reason and some because the authorities judged the parents to be incapable. What if someone thought the same of me? Or what if, God forbid, my disability caused me to have an accident and I accidentally hurt my child - would 'they' automatically take my baby from me? All of these thoughts haunted me, until I shared them with Corrine.

'Nobody is going to take your baby from you,' she said, reassuringly. 'We'll do everything possible to get you all the support you need, but nobody is going to take your baby away.' Corrine smiled at me as I struggled to hold back my tears. The pregnancy hormones were already taking hold of me!

Feeling reassured, I saw her out and then sighed with relief. I had worked myself up so much over nothing and now I had to really focus on not getting stressed, for my baby's sake. He or she needed me to be strong, especially as the next few months would present many more challenges, both emotional and physical.

Chapter 31

One strong, regular heartbeat

Over the next weeks, during quiet moments alone, I did start to wonder how I would manage all the challenges and demands of motherhood. I'm not afraid to admit that despite all my outward confidence, I was scared. Really scared.

I thought back to conversations with Mum and Dad, when they had voiced legitimate concerns about my becoming a parent. Whenever my nephews and niece threw a tantrum and were screaming the place down, they'd pointedly ask if I was taking note and that I should treasure life as it was. Although I knew that they only had my best interests at heart, nothing would squash my longing to be a Mum. My disability didn't rob me of those maternal instincts that most women felt, at one time or another.

Now, their warnings rang in my ears and on occasions, I began to panic. What if I couldn't manage? What if I brought this baby into the world, only to let the little mite down? How would I change a wriggly little baby who didn't understand my limitations? Would I be able to get out and about with my little one just like other mums? With all these questions weighing on my mind, I felt really scared. I searched the internet for stories from other disabled parents and although I found snippets of information, support for disabled parents seemed very limited.

Then I thought about the lady I had met in Reading, who was a brilliant mother in spite of her disability. Her daughter had gradually adapted to her needs and learnt how to help her Mum. Children are brilliant at adapting and I was sure that our baby would be too. Seeking further reassurance, I voiced my worries to Dean. 'We'll find ways for you to do things. Yes, it may take you longer, but at least you'll be able to do what you need to do.' Always the voice of reason, Dean stopped me worrying once again and my excitement at becoming a mum resumed.

A few weeks later, Mum and Dad arrived unexpectedly from Ireland. After they had moved back to Ireland, they brought a smaller house in Great Barr so that they could still come and go as they pleased. Their house is just around the corner from ours and they often turn up as a 'surprise', though I'm rarely surprised as they do this so often! On this particular occasion, I was sitting in our front room when Mum suddenly appeared at the window. Though I was pleased to see her, I was also very anxious. By this time, I was almost nine weeks pregnant and although I wasn't showing yet, I was worried Mum might guess. I felt guilty that I had such a big secret but I was not yet prepared to tell her and besides, I wanted Dad to be there too.

Mum stayed for a while, but I was on tenter hooks the whole time. As soon as she'd gone, I told Dean that now was our opportunity to share our news. We agreed to go round to their house the following evening. Although I was a grown, married woman, and I knew that this was the most normal, natural thing in the world, I still felt like an unruly teenager going home to confess that they'd accidentally fallen pregnant! I was so worried about Mum and Dad's reaction that I felt physically sick as we walked round to their house.

I had the conversation planned out in my head and it went something like this:

'There's something that we wanted to talk to you about.' Deep breath. 'You know, even before we got married that we were hoping to have a family and in March we went to see a Harley Street doctor. We wanted to talk to him about whether or not I was able to have a baby and what effect pregnancy might have on me.' I took out the letter from Mr O'Brien, which summarised everything he'd said during my appointment and I handed it to Mum. I gave her a few minutes to read it and then I knelt down beside the sofa where she and Dad were sat.

Another deep breath. Now or never. 'And the other good news is that I'm nine weeks pregnant!' My eyes glistened with tears and my voice began to break as I waited for their reaction. Much to my great relief, their tears joined mine as they hugged me and offered us both their congratulations. 'Well done Aideen, love,' Dad said, as he fought to contain tears.

'I knew the other night, didn't I say to you Jimmy?' Mum exclaimed, still clutching the letter and wiping away tears. A Mum's instinct I suppose! I think Mr O'Brien's letter had quietened some of their fears and they were genuinely happy and proud of me.

Once again, it was acknowledged that motherhood would present me with many challenges, but both Dean and I reassured Mum and Dad that we were fully prepared for what lay ahead of us and that no matter what, we'd find ways for me to do things. The conversation became much easier as talk turned towards my due date and the first scan in a few weeks' time. I began to relax as excitement crept in and it was a huge relief that despite their concerns, Mum and Dad were genuinely happy for us. They would be returning to Ireland in a few days and asked if I'd like to join them so that I could share my news with Collette, Martina and James. Although my scan wasn't for a few more weeks, I couldn't wait to tell them, so I jumped at the opportunity.

The walk home was much more relaxing and I knew that from now on, I'd be able to really enjoy my pregnancy and our preparations for parenthood. We still had lots of people to share our news with and I was looking forward to telling everyone else as soon as we'd had the reassurance of the first scan.

Though I was looking forward to it, I was also very nervous. At this stage, I didn't yet 'feel' pregnant (though a bout of morning sickness firmly told me I was!) I was scared that my body was playing tricks on me and that I wasn't really pregnant. I also had another concern. There were twins on both sides of the family and though I desperately wanted children, I wasn't sure how I'd cope with two at the same time. Dean kept joking about it, trying to wind me up, but I did fret about it. A lot.

My fears were quashed when the sonographer confirmed that there was just one, strong and regular heartbeat! Seeing our baby on the screen made everything so real and I couldn't wait to tell the world that I was going to be a mummy! As soon as we got home, I wheeled round to Mary to tell her the news. I simply said I had something to show her and watched her face as she looked at the scan picture and then ran over to hug me. She and her husband Joe were over the moon and Mary got straight on the phone to spread the news across Great Barr!

Our phone was permanently engaged that night as I excitedly rang family and friends. I never tired of saying the words, 'I'm going to be a mummy!', and waiting for the reaction. It was something I never dared to believe I would ever say and now, I intended to take every opportunity to say it!

Chapter 32
Morning, noon and night

Shortly after the first scan, we booked another appointment with Mr. O'Brien. At this stage, our intention was for me to have all my routine appointments and scans in Birmingham and then go to London for the birth, so that Mr. O'Brien could oversee the delivery. I know it sounds over the top, but I couldn't find another obstetrician with Mr. O'Brien's experience anywhere and he made me feel safe. I couldn't help but think about my own birth and I was absolutely terrified that history might repeat itself. I also knew that by going private, I was more likely to have the delivery that I wanted and receive one-to-one care during my labour.

Mr. O'Brien seemed to think differently. He reiterated what he had said during my first appointment. I wasn't at any more risk than any other woman giving birth and there was nothing to suggest that I needed specialist care. Even though he was effectively turning down business, he didn't think it was necessary for him to oversee my care, especially as he only practised in London. I had to agree that it seemed a little silly to travel up and down to London when it wasn't really necessary. Plus, Mr. O'Brien pointed out that being the second biggest city, Birmingham had some very experienced consultants and he was convinced that I'd be in good hands. Nonetheless, he was kind enough to give me his mobile number and told me to phone him if I had any concerns or questions. This being my first pregnancy, I was nervous and anxious but I trusted Mr. O'Brien's judgement and having his direct line reassured me immensely.

Around the time that I'd fallen pregnant, I had started to go to physiotherapy. I knew that the latter stages of my pregnancy would take a physical toll on me and both Dean and I wanted me to be as strong as possible so that I'd be able to maintain some level of mobility. I had an appointment every month and the physiotherapist gave me exercises to do on my own at home. When I was younger, I'd hated having to do my physio, but now I had more motivation. Although the exercises were tough, I just kept thinking of my baby and how I needed to be in the best possible health to give birth. In the following months, I was so glad that I'd made the effort.

There were some things that were beyond my control, mainly 'morning' sickness and heartburn. I say 'morning' sickness but it's not; it's 'morning, noon and night' sickness, and boy did I suffer! There were days when I could barely eat and in those moments, I would swear to Dean that this would be my first and only pregnancy! But again, the thought of my baby got me through it and eventually, the sickness passed.

It was Christmas by the time I started to show and I felt my baby move for the first time. It was so surreal, but such a wonderful feeling. Over the next few days and weeks, I often felt the baby move and it was always a lovely reassurance that all was well. I often thought how amazing it was that *I* was growing and nurturing this baby and how it turned out would be completely down to me. It was a frightening responsibility, but I took it seriously; I ate three square meals a day, every day and gave up everything that I was supposed to.

Shortly after Christmas, I had another scan and an opportunity to meet my consultant at Birmingham City Hospital. My mistrust in the medical profession surfaced again as I fretted over his response to me. I admit to being a bit hostile towards him, particularly after meeting someone as experienced and approachable as Mr. O'Brien. While he certainly didn't share the Irishman's charisma, Mr. Shah seemed to share his opinions, in that he saw no reason why I wouldn't be able to have a normal delivery, whatever that was!

I was pleased that I was being considered capable

of having a natural delivery and I really hoped and prayed that this would be the reality. But I wasn't yet convinced that I'd be able to cope with a normal delivery and Mr. Shah seemed reluctant to even discuss the possibility of a caesarean. He explained that the National Health Service operated a policy against planned caesarean sections unless there was a medical reason for it. Though I understood this, none of us yet knew how the pregnancy was going to affect me physically and I thought it was unfair to rule anything out at this stage.

Nonetheless, Mr. Shah did understand my anxiety so he decided to refer me to the Midwife Consultant. Her role was to oversee the care of vulnerable mothers or those with additional needs. As soon as I met her, I immediately felt reassured as she allowed me to talk through all of my concerns, including the possibility of history repeating itself. I felt tears welling up in my eyes as I explained what had happened at my birth and how I feared something bad happening to my baby. I knew deep down that I was being irrational, but it helped to voice my worries. The Midwife Consultant assured me that they would do everything possible to look after us both and that nearer the time, she would help me plan the birth and put everything I needed in place.

With my confidence in the NHS restored, I tried to concentrate on enjoying the rest of my pregnancy.

Dean and I picked out names and even though he begged me to, we decided against finding out the baby's sex. I really didn't mind what the baby was, as long as it was healthy, so I didn't see the point in finding out. Besides, I love surprises! As my pregnancy progressed and my bump slowly grew, I spent hours talking to the baby, willing it to keep growing and arrive safely. Little did I realise that I had a long way to go and a lot of anxiety to endure before that could happen.

Chapter 33

Not quite right

My pregnancy was going brilliantly and having finally overcome the morning sickness, I felt fantastic. Everybody kept asking me how I was and if I was still managing to walk. I'd proudly reply that I was still able to walk around the house and as yet, my growing bump wasn't causing me too many problems.

As Dean was busy with work, I tended to go and see the midwife on my own and then he would take a few hours off when I had appointments at the hospital. I was over half way through my pregnancy and attending a routine midwife appointment when we started to have cause for concern. My usual midwife was away and so another midwife was standing in for her. Everything seemed to be going well, until she measured my bump. 'That doesn't seem right.' She said with a puzzled and concerned look on her face. 'Let me just plot it on the graph.' I held my breath as she studied the graph and I searched her face for her conclusion.

'The baby doesn't seem to be growing, you need to

go to hospital for a scan.' She explained. The midwife had already checked the baby's heartbeat and it had been fine. I'd also felt the baby wriggling around that morning so I wasn't sure what was wrong. As the midwife got on the phone to the hospital, a million distressing thoughts whirled around my head. I heard the midwife arranging for me to go straight to the hospital and the urgency panicked me so much that I began to cry. I wished that I hadn't have come to the appointment on my own.

Once she'd hung up the phone, the midwife attempted to reassure me that everything would be fine and that the baby's heartbeat was strong. I was hardly able to speak so the midwife offered to phone Dean to explain what was happening. During the ten minute walk home, I tried to focus on the baby's heartbeat and keep as calm as I could. By the time I arrived, Dean had informed his boss of the situation and we were able to go straight to the hospital.

As we waited to be called in, I began to calm down slightly. At least if there was something wrong, I was now in the right place. Ever the pragmatist, Dean reasoned that the midwife hadn't seen me before and wasn't used to my movements so she had probably got the measurements wrong. I prayed that he was right.

The scan seemed to take ages and again, I searched the midwife's face for answers. Eventually, I quietly asked if everything was alright. I finally allowed myself to breathe when she replied that everything was fine. She went on to explain that there was a very slight slump in the baby's growth, but at this stage of the pregnancy it was insignificant and nothing to worry about. As a precaution, I would have to have another scan in two weeks, but the midwife stressed that it was normal after the scare that we'd had.

We went home reassured and I breathed a sigh of relief. Nonetheless, I couldn't help feeling anxious. I tried to relax and keep calm, I knew worrying would only stress the baby. Every kick and movement I felt was even more precious, as I knew the baby was doing well. And boy, did baby make its presence known! I'd frequently feel its little legs in my ribs and no moving about on my part would encourage the baby to switch position! Two weeks slowly passed and we returned to the hospital for another scan. Once again, we were reassured that the baby was well and that the growth was now considered normal again.

Over the next few weeks, there were yet more concerns about the size of my bump and the hospital felt like my second home. Each scan raised my anxiety levels and got me fretting that there was something wrong. We were at yet another scan when we discovered there *was* a problem. But not with the baby. We were told that the baby's measurements had been wrongly recorded at one of the previous scans and this had caused all the subsequent scans to be wrong. The baby was, and always had been, absolutely fine. I was so relieved, but also angry that I had been put through so much worry for nothing. It didn't fill me with confidence for the upcoming birth.

Nonetheless, the Midwife Consultant met with us again to make plans for when I finally had the baby. I'd already discussed pain relief with Mr. O'Brien. Though he had seen no reason why I wouldn't be able to have an epidural, I was concerned that my involuntary movements might make it difficult for it to be administered. Combine my spasms with the pain of labour and who could tell what kind of state I might be in! However, the Midwife Consultant arranged for me to meet the anaesthetist to see if it might be possible. To my great relief, he agreed that it would be possible and better still, that I could have it as soon as I was in established labour!

It was also arranged that I would have a private room on the ward and that despite normal visiting rules, Dean would be allowed to stay with me while I was in hospital. I'm not sure that Dean was as happy with this arrangement as I was, but I felt reassured that he'd be there if I needed him. I was worried that it might be more difficult to make myself understood during the labour so it was reassuring to know that Dean would be with me the whole time.

But as it turned out, he wasn't to be the only one by my side. Dean and I had talked about what to do when I went into labour and decided that it was probably best that we didn't tell anyone straight away. I didn't want people to worry, especially my Mum. I knew that like me, she'd be anxious and that my own birth would be preying on her mind. I reasoned that it would be better for us both if she wasn't with me. I worried about something going wrong and Mum being put through all the pain of my birth all over again. I knew she was worried and I desperately wanted to protect her, like she had always protected me.

With a week to go before my due date I was getting very anxious. I'd started reading every pregnancy forum I could find and had even brought some airy-fairy CD about 'Effective Birth Preparation', in an effort to keep myself calm. But nothing would soothe my anxieties. Then Mum and Dad turned up, as they often do from Ireland and though I love their visits, I'm not sure I've ever been as happy to see them walking up the drive! I almost cried as I greeted them, though I tried to hide it.

For the next ten days, I didn't have time for reading forums or listening to silly CDs. Mum kept me occupied and took my mind off my increasing pain and discomfort. We watched every game show that was on TV and wandered around the local shops, aimlessly. Anything to make the time go quicker.

Though I was still mobile, just about, it was becoming very difficult for me to get around and I often resorted to crawling around the house as the pressure on my pelvis became unbearable. As my due date came and went, there was no sign of baby despite my pleas to it to make an appearance soon!

My midwife was now visiting me at home as it was too difficult for me to get to the surgery, which was inaccessible with my wheelchair. She could see that things were getting too much for me and decided to try and get me booked in to be induced. But after examining me, my consultant rejected her request. Even though I was struggling physically, he saw no medical reason to induce me. In his view, I wasn't any different from any other woman who was a few days overdue. He explained to me and Mum that induction can cause complications so unless there was a very good reason, he wouldn't agree to it. Although I was physically exhausted and emotionally drained, I understood and respected his decision. I was pleased that I wasn't being treated any differently just because of my disability. After all, that's all I'd ever wanted.

Despite his conclusions, the doctor agreed to monitor me in a few days and it was during this appointment that he did a U-turn and decided on induction. Apparently, the baby's heartbeat dipped while I was hooked up to the monitor and although the baby was fine, it was considered best to induce me the next day.

   I was finally going to have my baby. I hardly slept that night with the nerves and excitement. I was finally going to become a mummy.

Chapter 34
Absolutely gorgeous

My bag had been packed for a month, in the hope that I might have the baby early. No such luck! This baby was quite happy to keep me waiting, however much discomfort that caused. After a restless night, the alarm finally sounded and we got ready to go to the hospital.

As we walked out to the car, my Dad was very conveniently walking the dog past our house. It was great to see a reassuring face when I was feeling so anxious, but as Dad hugged me and wished me luck, tears welled in my eyes again. So many emotions were whirling around inside and I was trying so hard to keep a lid on them. I didn't want Dad or Dean to know how anxious I really was, although I don't think I was that successful at hiding it. Dad kept it brief and I sensed he shared my anxiety.

All the way to the hospital, tears were never far away and I limited conversation for fear of losing control. I had to be brave for the baby's sake; breaking down now, before anything had even started, wasn't going to help either of us. I focused on the thought that when I returned home, it would be with our baby. I pushed away any thoughts of my own birth and focused on the day ahead.

As instructed, we arrived at the hospital at 8 am and were shown to a delivery suite to wait for a midwife. I should have known better than to expect anything to happen quickly. After all, this was the NHS. Staff popped in and out to do various things, but for the most part, we were left alone until lunchtime when I was finally induced. We were warned that it could take up to twenty-four, if not forty-eight hours for anything to happen so we settled in for what we thought would be a long wait.

One of the midwives came to monitor me, so I sent Dean to get himself something to eat. As we got chatting, the midwife asked me about my condition. As I explained that I had CP and how it had happened, I finally let my tears go. I confessed how frightened I was that something would go wrong and that although I knew I was being irrational, my biggest fear was history repeating itself. It was a relief to get things off my chest to someone who wasn't emotionally involved. The midwife held my hand and assured me that both me and the baby would be well looked after and that we were in good hands. After a good cry, I felt better and more ready to face what lay ahead.

By the time Dean returned, I was smiling again and willing the contractions to start. I didn't have to wait long. By 4 pm, just three hours after being induced, the pains started. So much for up to 48 hours! They were gradual and manageable to begin with, but then they stopped for a few hours! Mum phoned to see if it was alright to pop in and see me and by the time she arrived, my contractions were much stronger and much more frequent. As soon as I saw her, I knew that I didn't want her to leave me. She was only too delighted to stay with us and the banter between us all kept my mind off the pain. She kept me cool and chatted away to me as if we were just sitting watching TV and as soon as another contraction came, she reminded me to breathe and keep calm.

Nothing anyone tells you can prepare you for giving birth. During my pregnancy, I'd watched 'One Born Every Minute' every week, in the hope that I'd then know what I'd let myself in for. Mum used to laugh at me, but I wanted to at least *feel* prepared. I had consequently prepared myself for the worst pain imaginable and consoled myself that at least it was only for a relatively short period of time, hopefully. I'd only been in labour for a few hours when I felt the overwhelming need to push. But both Mum and the midwife kept telling me that I shouldn't as I was nowhere near ready. Trying to control that urge was a whole lot worse than the pain, I can tell you! Being my first baby, I had no idea what was going on, but Mum started to suspect that I was much further on than the consultant thought. I wasn't due to be examined for another few hours, but on Mum's advice, I requested that they examine me sooner.

In the meantime, the baby was being constantly monitored and the reassuring sound of the heartbeat was keeping me going. Everything was going really well until the midwife announced that she had lost the baby's heartbeat. I started to panic as she continued to try and find it again. There was suddenly talk of getting me ready for theatre and Mum helped me change into a hospital gown. Panic began to take over and I was convinced that this was my worst nightmare coming true. Dean and Mum kept as calm as they could and kept reassuring me that everything would be ok. After what seemed like an age, the midwife relaxed as she said she had located the baby's heartbeat again and that it was regular. Theatre had been avoided. For now.

I was finally examined and thrilled to be told that I was almost seven centimetres dilated. I had done most of the hard work without the epidural that I'd been promised. I was progressing much quicker than anyone had expected, especially as I'd been induced. The midwife arranged for the anaesthetist to come as soon as possible to administer the epidural. Already high on gas and air, I thanked him profusely for doing what was only his job as Mum held me as still as possible. I had been warned that it can sometimes take several attempts to get an epidural in. With my unpredictable movements, I was bracing myself for difficulties. I was amazed that the anaesthetist was successful first time and now hoped that the worst was over.

The epidural was starting to take effect and I was beginning to relax a bit more when the midwife announced that the baby's heartbeat had been lost again. This time, we couldn't afford to wait and before I knew what was happening, I was told to sign a consent form and then I was being whisked down to theatre. But nobody was telling me anything and I wasn't sure what I'd actually consented to. On my way to theatre, I remember asking the midwife if I was going to have a caesarean, but nobody was sure if that would be necessary until I got to theatre. Dean had gone to get changed so he could come into theatre with me and I was absolutely terrified that I was going to lose our baby.

As soon as I arrived in theatre and Dean was by my side, it was realised that I didn't need a caesarean and the surgeon would help the baby out with a ventouse. A ventouse, or vacuum extractor, is a cup-shaped instrument attached to the baby's head to assist the birth. Despite the epidural, I still knew when I needed to push and within a few minutes, at 5.41am on 28th June, our baby was born. It was a while before I heard a cry and I began to panic. But Dean could see much more than me and reassured me that the baby was just being checked over. It seemed like forever, but that first cry filled me with relief. I asked if the baby was a girl or boy but the staff wanted to show me. It was taking ages for them to bring him to us and I begged them to tell me. 'It's a boy!' one of the midwives announced.

We finally had our beautiful baby boy, Jack James Blackborough.

Every mother is biased about their children, but Jack was absolutely gorgeous and I couldn't take my eyes off him. I just couldn't believe that he was mine. As we lay in recovery waiting to be transferred to the ward, I thanked God that everything had gone well and that our baby was so perfect. The midwife asked if I'd like to try breast feeding and I eagerly agreed. I'd always wanted to breastfeed, but I'd heard so many negative experiences that I worried I'd have difficulty. But Dean was incredibly supportive and we agreed that I'd at least give it a really good try. I need not have worried at all. From that first feed, Jack just took to it and I soon felt equally as comfortable.

Visitors are not normally allowed in the recovery room, but my Dad arrived to take Mum home for some sleep and the midwife broke the rules to let Dad in for a few minutes. His face was a picture as he peered in to see Jack sleeping in his cot. 'That's another achievement ticked off the list, Aideen!' he said, smiling at me. Mum kept telling him how well I'd coped and I knew that despite their initial concerns, they were both so proud of me. It was wonderful for the five of us to spend those first few minutes together and I'll never forget it. Although tired and very groggy, I was on cloud nine.

The rest of the day passed in a blur of joyful phone calls, sleep and pure elation. As had been promised, we were put in a private room with an en suite so we had peace and privacy. Like most newborns, Jack was content to sleep off the trauma of being born into a whole new world, giving me an opportunity to also recover. Every time I woke up, I'd gaze over at Jack with tears in my eyes and thank God again for such a perfect little boy. Dean spent the first night with us and we began to bond as a family. Still numb and unable to move much, I wasn't able to do anything for Jack except of course, breast feed him. When Dean went home for a rest, I was reliant on the staff to help me lift and change Jack. While I knew that I should concentrate on my recovery, I still felt frustrated and useless. I was anxious to start doing more for Jack, partly to reassure myself that I was capable of taking care of him. On the Sunday, I felt much better so I begged to be discharged. I knew that once I got home and was comfortable in my own environment, I would be able to find my own ways of doing things. I was over the moon to be discharged that afternoon.

It wasn't long before I was hesitantly changing my first nappy, with Dean by my side for much needed reassurance. Little did I realise that these early days, before Jack learnt to wriggle and roll over, were to be the easiest! These days, I'm lucky if I can get his nappy off before he tries to escape and it can be really difficult to change him without Dean's help. Even if I do manage to get a clean nappy on him, it's often lopsided and in danger of falling off. Like most babies, nappy changes just aren't on Jack's agenda and it's a problem that I've pondered for a long time. Now as Jack approaches potty training stage, we've started to use pull-ups, which are much easier. Even though Jack still resists being changed, he doesn't seem to mind me putting on his 'big boy pants' quite as much as a nappy.

Still a little sore and very unsteady on my feet after the birth, I relied on Dean to lift and carry Jack wherever I needed him to be. As my confidence began to grow, I'd sit on the edge of the sofa, tuck my hands securely under Jack's arms and when I was certain that I had a good grip, I'd carefully lift Jack up into my arms when he needed a feed. I soon learnt that holding a hungry baby while trying to undo a maternity bra was no easy task, so I'd get myself ready for feeding and then pick him up. Once I'd mastered this, I took the next step and began laying a sleepy

Jack back down in his Moses basket, all the while trying to control the shakiness in my arms, so that I wouldn't wake him, and support his head as I lay him down.

I was constantly thinking about the best ways for me to do things independently so that I wouldn't have to rely on Dean quite so much. One day, when Jack was a few weeks old, I was in the living room with him and I wanted to go into the kitchen. There was nobody else around so it was a good opportunity to try something without feeling self-conscious. Jack was lying in his Moses basket so I knelt beside it and gently pushed it across the floor, 'walking' on my knees towards the kitchen. The first time I did it, Jack's face was a picture, as if to say, 'Where are we going, Mummy?' It worked really well, even if I did wear holes in all of my jeans! Jack was safe and I felt confident and that was all that mattered. That became my way of getting him from A to B in those early days and I was proud and also relieved that I was finding my own ways of doing things, even if they were a bit unconventional. Friends and family would come to visit and I think many of them were surprised by how well I was managing, but I was just taking care of my son the best way I knew. In those early days, I was reluctant to accept offers of help, always eager to prove to people and more importantly, to myself, that I could look after Jack.

Although my confidence was constantly growing, I

also knew that I still needed someone to be on hand to help me, just in case. Although I knew that I was totally capable of caring for Jack, I felt much more confident knowing that Dean was around, should I ever get into difficulty. We'd initially agreed that Dean would have six weeks off work to spend with us and we began to think about and discuss the support that I'd need once he went back to work. We thought about employing a full-time nanny and personal assistant, who could also help me with household chores. However, given the fact that Dean could be out at work for up to twelve hours a day, we knew that finding the right person would be both tricky and expensive. I was able to do almost everything for Jack so it seemed that we'd be paying someone just to be on hand, 'in case'.

Then it dawned on us. The money that we'd use to pay a nanny could be used to keep Dean at home and while he'd be around if I needed him, he could also work on his own development project. We both have businesses that we wanted to build up, so we could share the childcare and both work. It was the perfect solution!

Once we'd decided on this option, we settled into a routine where I worked each morning and Dean worked in the afternoon. We both had quality time with Jack and as time went by, we were able to share the joy as Jack reached new milestones.

But one such happy event, to officially register Jack, was ruined by a rude and ignorant registrar. It was an occasion which I was looking forward to, as I'm sure all new parents do. However, my excitement and pride was soon replaced by upset and anger when we entered the registrar's office. With Jack wriggling and crying in my arms, she turned to ask me my name but as soon as I opened my mouth, she looked at me blankly, making it clear she couldn't understand me and then immediately turned to my Dean, expecting him to speak for me. As I've said before, I have a speech impairment, but with time and a little patience, it isn't difficult to understand me. After all, I wouldn't be a successful trainer if I couldn't communicate effectively!

From then on, she directed all questions to Dean and although he told her she was being ignorant, she completely ignored him and continued directing all her questions at him. I continued to try to interject, telling the registrar that I was quite capable of answering her questions, but she then bluntly stated that only one parent was required to register Jack. In other words, despite being Jack's mum, I was surplus to requirements.

I was absolutely fuming, but unfortunately Jack was very unsettled and in need of a feed so it wasn't an appropriate time to challenge her ignorance and I left Dean to complete the process while I tended to Jack. I was angry and frustrated at being made to feel like this just because the registrar was too ignorant to take the time to listen to me. She ruined an important occasion, one which I can never repeat and yet she was completely oblivious of this fact.

As I fought to contain both my anger and my tears, I wondered how many more similar experiences would challenge me as a disabled parent. Just as I'd always fought against disability discrimination, I felt like I'd always have to prove that my disability wasn't a barrier to be being a good parent. But whatever anyone else thought or said, I made a whispered promise to Jack: that I'd always be the best mummy to him, no matter what obstacles I might face.

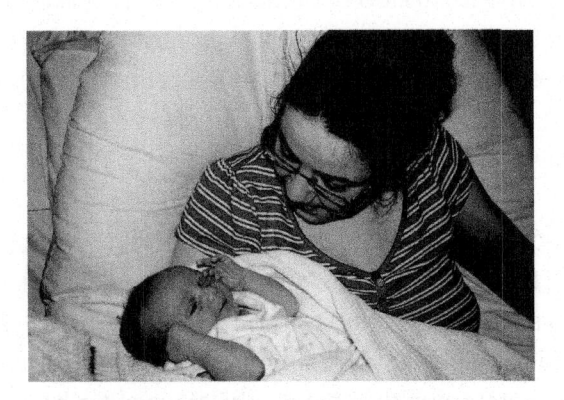

I just couldn't believe that Jack was *my* little boy

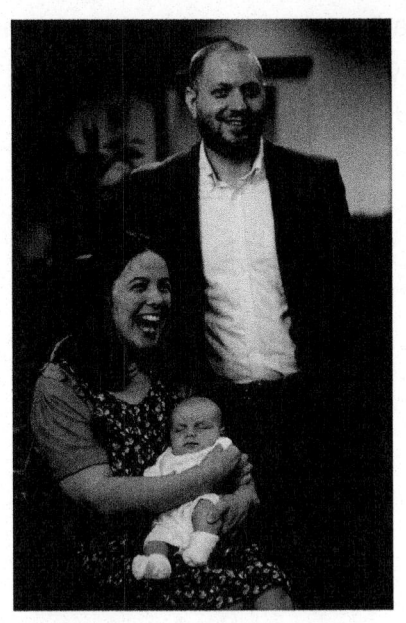

Having Dean at home helped build my confidence as I found the best ways for me

Chapter 35
We'll see!

As Jack got bigger, new challenges began to present themselves. I wanted to be able to take Jack out and about by myself but a wheelchair and a pushchair don't exactly mix well! So we went shopping for a harness and/or a sling so I could carry Jack on my lap. Although there were lots of different ones available, they weren't exactly easy for me to use.

The sling initially seemed like the best option, in that it was easy for me to put on, but it wasn't easy to get Jack in a comfortable position. I used it a couple of times, but I never felt one hundred percent confident with it. While the harness felt much more secure, there were lots of clips and buckles to contend with and I still wasn't able to independently attach Jack to me. Dean was happy to help whenever I wanted to go out, but I never strayed too far, just in case Jack needed a nappy change. We went round to visit Mary Mac or my parents, who soon became adept at securing Jack into his harness and attaching him to me. Dad called him my little Joey and I was as proud as punch being able to take him out and show him off.

As Jack piled on the pounds, the harness became too tight on him and I wondered what would be my next option. As I'd already discovered, there was very little information for disabled parents and even less adapted equipment to help solve such problems. We brought another harness, usually used for toddlers who want to walk alongside their parents, thinking we could hook my wheelchair seatbelt around it but I found that Jack was able to move around quite a bit. Unless I was constantly able to hold him with my non-driving hand, he just didn't feel secure. So there was nothing else for it except to extend my wheelchair seatbelt around us both. It seems to work well for the relatively short trips that I make with Jack, but until he's able to walk safely alongside me, I can't really take him when I go shopping as I need my lap to hold a basket and my spare hand to reach for things. I sometimes think that being an octopus would solve many of my motherhood challenges!

It certainly would have helped when we started Jack on solids. I find it difficult enough feeding myself sometimes, so I was somewhat apprehensive when I began trying to feed Jack. Always eager for his food, Jack would become impatient as I attempted to load the spoon and then get it safely to his mouth. If I was lucky, some of it would reach its intended destination. If not, one of two things would happen: I'd either start shaking and drop the food or, eager to help, Jack would grab the spoon and send its contents flying! In either case, it ended with both Jack and I being frustrated and I'd ask Dean to step in and help.

After a few failed attempts at feeding Jack, I became anxious and tearful, as I felt like I was failing my baby. Up until now, I'd always found a way to do things and I was able to do everything that he needed. I consoled myself with the fact that I was still breast feeding him and that was the one thing I could do for him that no-one else could. Always supportive, Dean encouraged me to persevere with feeding him solids and decided to look online for spoons which might be easier for me to grip. I was sceptical that anything could make a difference, after all, it was my spasms which were ultimately the problem and there was little that could be done about those. But never a defeatist, I agreed that anything was worth a try.

Dean brought spoons which were designed for kids who were just learning to feed themselves. They were quite chunky and had a much shorter handle than the ones that I'd been using, so I had much more control. The spoon itself was more curved, making it easier to keep food in place. To my surprise, they made a huge difference and my confidence was quickly restored. 'You see, there isn't anything that can't be solved, we just have to think about things a bit more laterally,' Dean said and with his reassurance, I knew that I'd always find a way to do whatever I needed to.

Another difficulty was getting Jack in and out of his cot. The Moses basket had been relatively easy once I'd built up my confidence, because I could kneel beside it and lift Jack in and out. I was nowhere near as confident lifting him while standing and I worried about how I'd jump this next hurdle. We brought a cot which had collapsing sides, thinking that this would help, but as soon as it arrived, we realised that the sides only collapsed with the mattress in its lowest position. This meant that it was of little help, as I'd still need to reach quite a way into the cot to pick Jack up. Just after buying the cot, we found one online which had a gate in the middle, which would have meant I could have knelt on the floor and picked Jack up, but as we had already bought one, it was too late. Something to archive for the future perhaps?

While Jack was in our room, I could kneel on our bed and get him out, but it was too difficult to get him into the cot if he was sleeping, as he often was after his bed time feed. It became our routine for me to take my mobile up to bed and when I'd finished feeding and Jack was fast asleep, I'd give Dean one ring and he'd come up and lay Jack down in the cot. As soon as Jack moved into his own room, our routine changed. I'd do his last feed downstairs and then Dean would carry him up to bed. It sometimes upset and frustrated me that I couldn't put him to bed, but I knew that would change as he got older. Indeed, he can now walk, run and climb the stairs, so I'm able to follow him up and then sit on a chair beside his cot while I lift him into it.

His nappy changes can still be troublesome and frustrating as Jack wriggles and rolls all over the place, eager to get on with the things that are on *his* agenda! I have a few tricks that help keep him still such as producing an interesting toy or even a bottle! But as I've mentioned, failing everything else, I've found that pull-ups are much easier to get on than nappies, even if I have to chase Jack around the room to get them on!

Of course, I can never say that I wasn't warned about how demanding motherhood would be and I've faced many additional challenges. My problem solving skills are constantly being tested, that's for sure! But I only have to look at Jack and see his little arms reach out for me to know that it is absolutely worth it. When I creep into his room at night just to watch him sleeping peacefully, I thank God for my beautiful little boy. Despite the many difficulties and challenges, being a mum truly is the most rewarding job in the world.

In the days and weeks after Jack's arrival, I swore that Jack would be an only child. The latter months of my pregnancy had been so difficult and I wasn't sure if I would be able to do it again. The fear of being rushed to theatre during labour and not knowing if my baby would be okay had scared me to the core. That and I wasn't yet sure if the challenges of motherhood would prove too much. But as the weeks turned into months and I watched Jack growing and truly thriving, I realised that I'd done it. I was his Mummy and he didn't care that I had CP, it was totally irrelevant. The love that we shared was unconditional and always would be.

Now that Jack is a toddler, people sometimes ask me when number two will be arriving. My previous hesitation is gone and with a twinkle in my eye, I just smile and say, 'We'll see!'

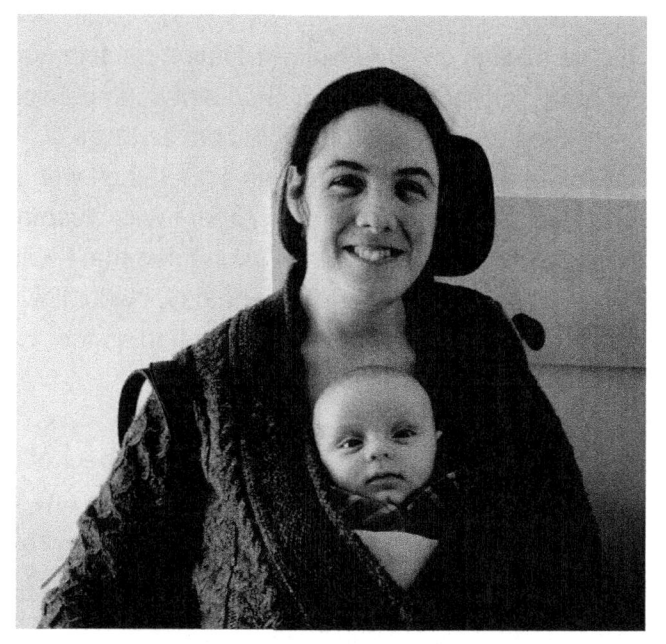

With time and thought, I found solutions for the problems that being a disabled parent presented

Afterword

I've always enjoyed writing. During my final year of primary school, I entered a short story competition and surprised myself by winning first prize. I was absolutely delighted; there was something I was really good at and it didn't matter whether I was disabled or not. So when a family friend suggested that I write my life story, I promised her that one day, I would! Almost twenty years later, I finally felt like I had a story worthy of telling. Thanks Jenny!

I see my disability as a very positive aspect of who I am; I don't let it define, control or limit me in any way. However, over the years, there have been several people who have tried to hold me back, not believing that I could achieve anything worthwhile. There have been authority figures who doubted my ability to cope with mainstream education. There have been bullies who have picked on me for walking a bit funny. There have also been employers who have discriminated against me because they believed their clients wouldn't understand somebody with a speech impediment. Every day, I've faced new challenges and experienced every possible emotion in overcoming them.

Despite my disability, I've achieved almost everything that I've put my mind to and that's the main reason why I wrote this book. To show that disabled people are just as capable as anyone else and that if you're determined enough, anything is possible.

When I was born, my parents knew very little about cerebral palsy. They just had to take every day as it came. From the day that I was diagnosed, my Mum and Dad have wanted me to be treated just like anyone else. Their supportive, positive attitude has inspired me to aim high and achieve things which other people believed were beyond my capabilities. Having a disabled child is scary and that's one reason why I wanted to share my story; I hope it will inspire parents of disabled children to push for what they think is right for their child, as my parents did.

As a disabled business woman, a wife and a mum, life is a challenge; there have been highs and lows, but with a loving family and some wonderful friends, I'm living my life to the maximum. I'll say it again: I have cerebral palsy; *it* doesn't have me.

I hope that you've enjoyed reading this book as much as I've enjoyed writing it.

Aideen Blackborough
July 2015

Printed in Great Britain
by Amazon